Preparatory Manual of
Pathology

for Medical Laboratory Technology Students

Preparatory Manual of
Pathology
for Medical Laboratory Technology Students

Sonam Kumar Pruthi

MBBS, MD (Pathology)

Specialist
Department of Pathology
NDMC Medical College and
Hindu Rao Hospital, Delhi

Namrata Sarin

MBBS, MD (Pathology)

Professor and Head
Department of Pathology
NDMC Medical College and
Hindu Rao Hospital, Delhi

Sompal Singh

MBBS, MD (Pathology), MBA (Hospital Admn), BSc (Statistics)

Senior Specialist
Department of Pathology
Hindu Rao Hospital, Delhi

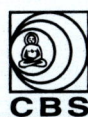

CBS

CBS Publishers & Distributors Pvt Ltd

New Delhi • Bengaluru • Chennai • Kochi • Kolkata • Mumbai
Bhopal • Bhubaneswar • Hyderabad • Jharkhand • Nagpur • Patna • Pune • Uttarakhand • Dhaka (Bangladesh)

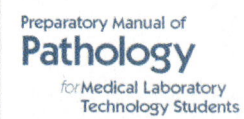

Preparatory Manual of
Pathology
for **Medical Laboratory Technology Students**

ISBN: 978-93-88178-94-5

First Edition: 2019

Published by Satish Kumar Jain and produced by Varun Jain for
CBS Publishers & Distributors Pvt Ltd
4819/XI Prahlad Street, 24 Ansari Road, Daryaganj, New Delhi 110 002, India.
Ph: 23289259, 23266861, 23266867   Fax: 011-23243014   Website: www.cbspd.com
e-mail: delhi@cbspd.com; cbspubs@airtelmail.in.

Corporate Office: 204 FIE, Industrial Area, Patparganj, Delhi 110 092
Ph: 4934 4934   Fax: 4934 4935   e-mail:publishing@cbspd.com;
publicity@cbspd.com

Branches

- **Bengaluru:** Seema House 2975, 17th Cross, K.R. Road, Banasankari 2nd Stage, Bengaluru 560 070, Karnataka
  Ph: +91-80-26771678/79   Fax: +91-80-26771680   e-mail: bangalore@cbspd.com
- **Chennai:** 7, Subbaraya Street, Shenoy Nagar, Chennai 600 030, Tamil Nadu
  Ph: +91-44-26260666, 26208620   Fax: +91-44-42032115   e-mail: chennai@cbspd.com
- **Kochi:** 42/1325, 1326, Power House Road, Opp KSEB Power House, Ernakulam 682 018, Kochi, Kerala
  Ph: +91-484-4059061-65   Fax: +91-484-4059065   e-mail: kochi@cbspd.com
- **Kolkata:** No. 6/B, Ground Floor, Rameswar Shaw Road, Kolkata-700014 (West Bengal), India
  Ph: +91-33-2289-1126, 2289-1127, 2289-1128   e-mail: kolkata@cbspd.com
- **Mumbai:** 83-C, Dr E Moses Road, Worli, Mumbai-400018, Maharashtra
  Ph: +91-22-24902340/41   Fax: +91-22-24902342   e-mail: mumbai@cbspd.com

Representatives

• Bhopal	0-8319310552	• Bhubaneswar	0-9911037372
• Hyderabad	0-9885175004	• Jharkhand	0-9811541605
• Nagpur	0-9021734563	• Patna	0-9334159340
• Pune	0-9623451994	• Uttarakhand	0-9716462459
• Dhaka (Bangladesh)	01912-003485		

Printed at   Goyal Offset Printers, GT Karnal Road, Industrial Area, Delhi, India

to
my loved ones

Foreword

D r Sonam Kumar Pruthi was a dedicated postgraduate student during his MD (Pathology) training-cum-tutorship in Kasturba Medical College, Mangalore, Manipal Academy of Higher Education (MAHE). It is my esteemed pleasure as well as a proud moment for me as his teacher and dear friend to write the Foreword to his book *Preparatory Manual of Pathology for Medical Laboratory Technology Students*.

In this well thought of endeavor to make academics easier for the trainees of medical laboratory technology (MLT), Dr Sonam researched to understand the requirement of a worthwhile learning aid for these students. In consultation with these trainees and his peers he realized that there was no simple, user-friendly and comprehensive pathology laboratory manual for the undergraduate MLT trainee students. The students had to refer to voluminous textbooks, study material of various correspondence courses, notes passed on by their seniors which were riddled with inaccuracies, and manuals which mention obsolete tests or were not updated timely. He then undertook an uphill task to study the curriculum, examination papers and training program of diploma and bachelor courses of MLT of various universities, and understand their commonalities, requirements of the theory and practical examinations, and expectations of the job market.

This book has 84 chapters, which encompasses histotechniques, cytotechniques, laboratory practices in clinical pathology and hematology, and technical aspects of transfusion medicine and immunohematology. To top it all, quality assurance and managerial issues have also been adequately dealt with in this book. Since this book is essentially a preparatory manual, each chapter has been elucidated under headings and sub-headings in a point-wise format so that the student can easily read and revise the content. The highlight of the book is its lucid language, simple flowcharts, color diagrams and microphotographs in each section. This beautifully drafted learning aid is definitely going to fill the void of a good preparatory manual of laboratory techniques in pathology and the students will be truly benefitted.

Dr Sonam is a voracious reader and hardworking researcher. Coupled with his passion to teach and intractable love for pathology, he has been able to accomplish the commendable feat of completing his fourth book within five years of completing postgraduate training. His other three books are *Comprehensive Review of Pathology, Preparatory Manual of Pathology for Undergraduate Students* and *My Pathology Notes for FMGE* have all been good sellers and received well by the students throughout the country.

My heartfelt best wishes to Dr Pruthi in this venture and may God bless him with continuing success.

Shrijeet Chakraborti
MD, DNB, PDF (Neuropath), PGDEA, MNAMS
Specialty Doctor (Histopathology), Leighton Hospital, Crewe
Mid Cheshire Hospitals, NHS Foundation Trust, Cheshire, United Kingdom
Ex-Associate Professor and In-Charge, Blood Bank
Department of Pathology, Kasturba Medical College, Mangalore
Manipal Academy of Higher Education (MAHE), India

Preface

The purpose of writing this book
In our hospital, we conduct three years professional course for BSc medical laboratory technology students. After discussion with our college students and while listening to their queries, we came to know about the vast course for their professional examinations and also learnt that there is no single book that covers all important topics for their professional examinations. We also learnt, that students have to refer to multiple books and also search online for covering different topics for their examinations. We promised them of writing a single book that will cover all major sections of their examinations related to our practising subject.

How did we write this book?
Book is written according to the university syllabus and what is being asked in BSc (MLT) professional examinations. We have referred to the detailed syllabus provided by the University for students professional examinations and also have gone through the last few years university examination question papers, in order to learn the pattern of examination and questions being asked.

Why should you read this book?
Book is divided into six sections, i.e. 1. Hematology, 2. Histological Techniques including stains, 3. Histopathology and Cytology, 4. Laboratory Management, 5. Clinical Pathology and 6. Transfusion Medicine. It is written, keeping in mind that it will be read by students, who have just finished their schooling, thus the language has been kept very simple, and content written point-wise. Also numerous flowcharts, diagrams and figures, wherever required, have been added in order to make the text easy to understand. Beautiful colours have been used for writing the text which also makes the book attractive to read and easy to recall. The content provided in each chapter is adequate as per the course demand and the student should be well-versed of the same to do well in examinations.

How one should go about this book?
Nothing is achieved easy and in medical field, constant upgradation of knowledge is required. This book also has been written keeping the same in mind. One reading will never make you learn and remember all the facts of this book. Constant efforts should be made by the students for repetitive revisions, and to be thorough with the subject. Thus, multiple revisions of the book holds the key to score good marks.

Also, many students will be preparing and applying for future professional courses like MSc in different medical streams. Facts learnt from this book will help the students to prepare for their entrance examinations and will also help the students practise the technical aspects of laboratory medicine in the best possible way.

Wishing you all the best for your good future.

Valuable suggestions, if any, to improve the book, are always welcome!

Sonam Kumar Pruthi
Namrata Sarin
Sompal Singh

Acknowledgments

We would like to express our gratitude towards our teachers, students and colleagues, whose guidance and motivation helped us to write and finish this book.

We also want to thank our family for their unconditional love and immense support, which cannot be exemplified with words.

We would also like to thank Ms Shakti Kalani, Mr Sukhwinder Singh, and Mr Santosh Sharma, Hindu Rao Hospital, for providing me Medical Laboratory Technology course details and their valuable opinion for framing of this book.

We would also like to thank Mr YN Arjuna, Senior Vice President—Publishing, Editorial and Publicity, CBS Publishers & Distributors, and his editorial team for their constant hard work, which made publication of this book possible.

Sonam Kumar Pruthi
Namrata Sarin
Sompal Singh

Contents

Section III: Histopathology and Cytology

Section IV: Laboratory Management

Section V: Clinical Pathology

Section VI: Transfusion Medicine

Section I

Hematology

Chapters

Red Blood Cells and Anemia

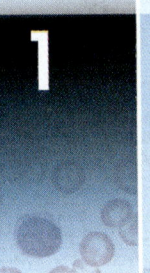

RED BLOOD CELL

- RBC is 7–8 microns in size, appears round with smooth contours and stain deep pink at the periphery and paler in the center.
- Central pallor is one-third of the diameter of the RBC.

Function

Transport and delivery of oxygen to the tissues.

RBC Count

- RBC range for men is 4.7 to 6.1 million cells per microliter
- RBC range for non-pregnant women is 4.2 to 5.4 million cells per microliter.

Morphology

a. *Normal RBC* is normocytic (normal size) normochromic (normal staining intensity)
b. *RBCs with abnormal size*
   - Microcytes (small RBCs)
   - Macrocytes (large RBCs)
c. *RBCs with varying hemoglobin content*
   - Hypochromic (RBCs with increased area of central pallor)
   - Dimorphic (two distinct populations exist together, e.g. microcytic and macrocytic RBCs)
d. *RBCs with variation in shape*
   - Sickle cells (RBC with both ends pointed and sickle shaped)

- Spherocytes (small RBCs show absence of central one-third of pallor)
- Schistocytes (fragmented RBCs)
- Target cells (RBCs with a central stained area and a peripheral stained rim with unstained cytoplasm in-between)

e. *RBC inclusions*
   - Basophilic stippling (presence of numerous, basophilic granules in the RBCs)
   - Howell-Jolly bodies (nuclear remnants situated peripherally on RBCs)
   - Pappenheimer bodies (basophilic, small, iron containing granules in RBCs)
   - Cabot's ring (figure of 8 appearing structure on RBC)

f. *Immature RBCs*
   - Polychromatophils (young RBC with RNA material within themselves)
   - Nucleated RBCs (erythroblasts)

g. *RBC arrangement*: Rouleaux formation: RBCs appear as stack of coins, being present on top of one another.

ANEMIA

A. Iron Deficiency Anemia

Due to reduced iron in body, there occurs reduced hemoglobin synthesis.

Peripheral Smear (Fig. 1.1)

- RBCs are microcytic (small size) and hypochromic (more than one-third of central pallor of the RBC) in chronic cases.
- Mild to moderate anisocytosis (change in cell size) and poikilocytosis (change in cell shape)
- Platelets can be normal/increased

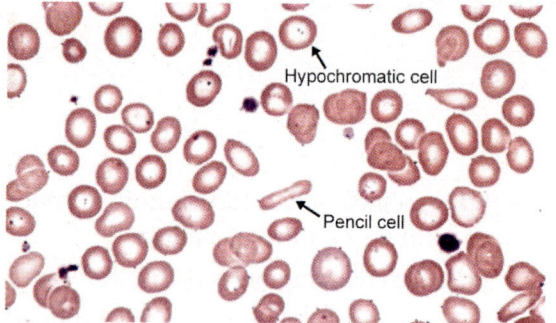

Fig. 1.1: Peripheral smear of iron deficiency anemia

B. Megaloblastic Anemia

- Occurs due to impairment of DNA synthesis and defective nuclear maturation.
- This results in nuclear to cytoplasmic asynchrony.

Peripheral Smear (Fig. 1.2)

- Shows macro-ovalocytes (large RBCs, which are oval in shape)
- Shows megaloblasts and hypersegmented neutrophils (containing 5 lobes in >5% neutrophils or containing 6 or more lobes)

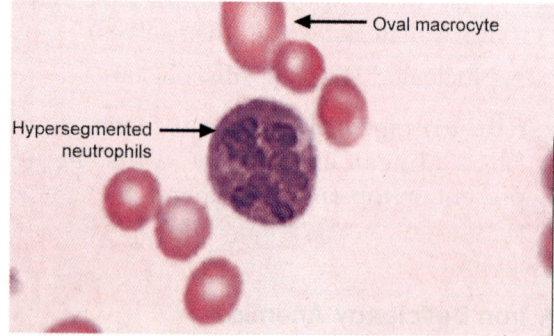

Fig. 1.2: Smear showing features of macrocytic anemia

- Can show red blood cells with multiple Howell-Jolly bodies (nuclear remnants present at the periphery of RBC)
- Reticulocyte count is low

C. Thalassemia

- Hemoglobin is composed of alpha and beta chains
- Deletion of these chains results in α-thalassemia and β-thalassemia.

Peripheral Smear (Fig. 1.3)

- Microcytic hypochromic RBCs
- Target cells, fragmented RBCs, nucleated RBCs, basophilic stippling and Howell-Jolly bodies (Fig. 1.4).

D. Sickle Cell Anemia

- Point mutation in β-globin gene leads to replacement of glutamate residue with a valine residue.

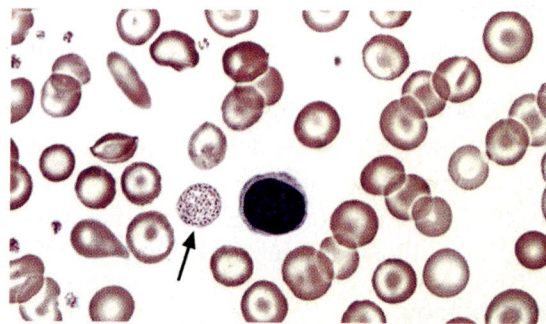

Fig. 1.3: RBCs showing microcytes, anisopoikilo-cytosis, target cells, basophilic stippling (arrow)

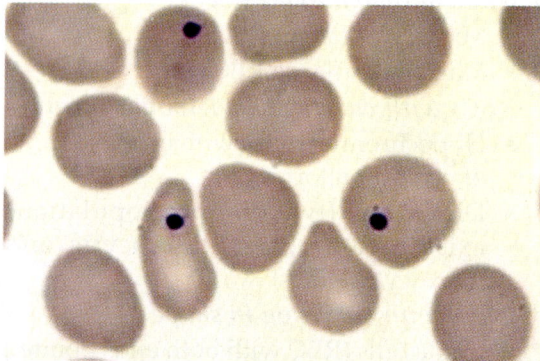

Fig. 1.4: Howell-Jolly bodies

- Results in abnormal RBC production, which when undergoes de-oxygenation becomes sickle shaped.

Peripheral Smear (Fig. 1.5)

- Sickle shaped RBCs
- Polychromatophilic RBCs
- Target cells, Howell-Jolly bodies

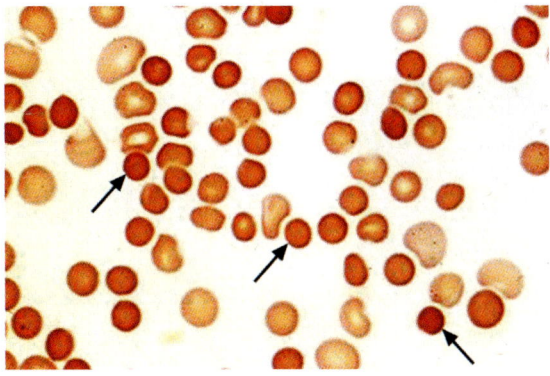

Fig. 1.6: Spherocytes in hereditary spherocytosis (arrows)

- RBCs appear small and lack central pallor (microspherocytes)
- Increased reticulocyte count

F. Glucose-6-Phosphatase Deficiency

- Occurs due to enzyme glucose-6-phosphatase dehydrogenase (G6PD) deficiency.
- Results in destruction of RBCs in the spleen and blood.

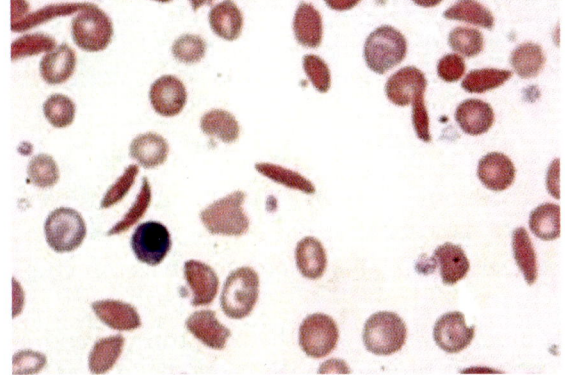

Fig. 1.5: Sickle shaped RBCs and a single nucleated (n) RBC

E. Hereditary Spherocytosis

- Occurs due to RBC membrane defect
- Defective red cell membrane components, i.e. α-spectrin, β-spectrin, ankyrin, band 4.2, or band 3 are seen.
- These mutations lead to red cells to lose membrane fragments.

Peripheral Smear (Fig. 1.6)

- Microcytic hypochromic anemia

Peripheral Smear (Fig. 1.7)

- Polychromatic RBCs
- Heinz bodies (appear as dark inclusions in RBCs)
- Bite cells, which occur due to splenic removal of denatured hemoglobin.
- Splenic macrophages remove these Heinz bodies and RBCs now are called "bite cells".

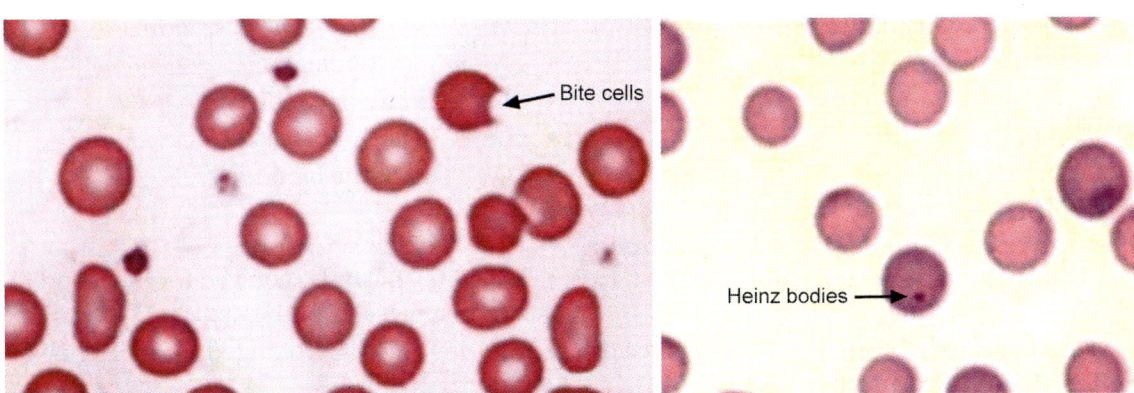

Fig. 1.7: Bite cells and Heinz bodies in G6PD deficiency smear

Laboratory Tests in Bleeding Disorders

1. BLEEDING TIME

- Assesses primary hemostasis
- Dependent on functioning of platelets and blood vessels
- A superficial skin puncture or incision is made and the time required for bleeding to stop is measured.
- Assessment is done by Ivy's method

Ivy's Method

Principle: With the help of lancet blades, three punctures are made on the dorsal surface of forearm under standard pressure, and the average time required for blood to stop oozing out from the puncture site is noted.

Equipment

- Sphygmomanometer
- Sterile disposable lancet blades (2–2.5 mm blade)
- Stop watch
- Filter paper

Methods

- A sphygmomanometer cuff is wrapped around the upper arm and inflated to 40 mm of Hg.
- Dorsal surface of forearm is cleaned with 70% ethanol and allowed to dry.
- Three punctures are made (about 5 cm apart) with lancet blade, one after an another.
- A stop watch is started as soon as puncture is made.
- Blood oozing from the puncture wound is gently blotted with a filter paper at 15 seconds interval.
- Timer is stopped, when blood no longer stains the filter paper.
- Time required for bleeding to cease from all the three puncture wounds is noted.
- Average time should be taken and is reported as bleeding time.
- Puncture site is covered with a sterile adhesive strip.

Result

Reference range: 2–7 minutes.

Prolonged bleeding time is seen in

- Thrombocytopenia
- Platelet function disorders
- von Willebrand disease
- Disorders of the blood vessels

2. CLOTTING TIME

- Measures the time required for the blood to clot in a glass test tube kept at 37°C.
- Clotting time is prolonged in deficiency of clotting factor.

ASSESSED BY CAPILLARY TUBE METHOD AND LEE-WHITE METHOD

a. Capillary Tube Method

Requirements

Pricking needle, stopwatch, glass capillary tube (10 cm long), cotton swab, alcoholic swab.

Methods

- Apply alcoholic cotton swab on the fingertip. Allow it to dry naturally.
- Prick the finger, immediately stopwatch is started.
- Dip one end of the capillary tube on the drop of blood.
- Allow to fill the capillary tube with blood
- After every 30 seconds, with the use of stop watch, break a small piece of capillary.
- Repeat breaking at regular time intervals, till fibrin thread appears at the broken end of capillary tube.
- Record time intervals between fingerprick and appearance of the fibrin thread at the broken ends of capillary tube and that is called the clotting time of blood.

b. Lee-White Method

Requirements

Water bath at 37°C, test tubes, stopwatch, syringes, fresh whole blood.

Methods

- Three-labeled glass test tubes labeled with patient's name are taken and numbered as 1, 2, and 3.
- Venepuncture is performed using a 20-gauge needle and 4 ml of blood is drawn.
- Remove the needle from the syringe, and fill each of the three tubes with 1 ml blood.
- Last 1 ml of blood is discarded
- Start the stopwatch as soon as the blood enters the syringe.
- Place the three test tubes in 37°C water bath
- At exactly 3 min, remove the first tube from water bath and tilt gently to a 45° angle to see whether the blood has clotted.

- If the blood is not clotted, return it to the water bath and examine it at 30 seconds intervals.
- After the blood in the first tube has clotted, examine the second tube immediately.
- Then examine the 3rd tube.
- Record the time it took the blood in the 3rd test tube to clot.

Result

Normal clotting time: 2 to 9 minutes.

3. PROTHROMBIN TIME (PT)

Assesses the coagulation factors in extrinsic pathway (factor VII) and common pathway (factor X, V, prothrombin, fibrinogen).

Principle (Fig. 2.1)

Tissue thromboplastin and calcium are added to plasma and clotting time is determined.

Equipment

- Water bath at 37°C

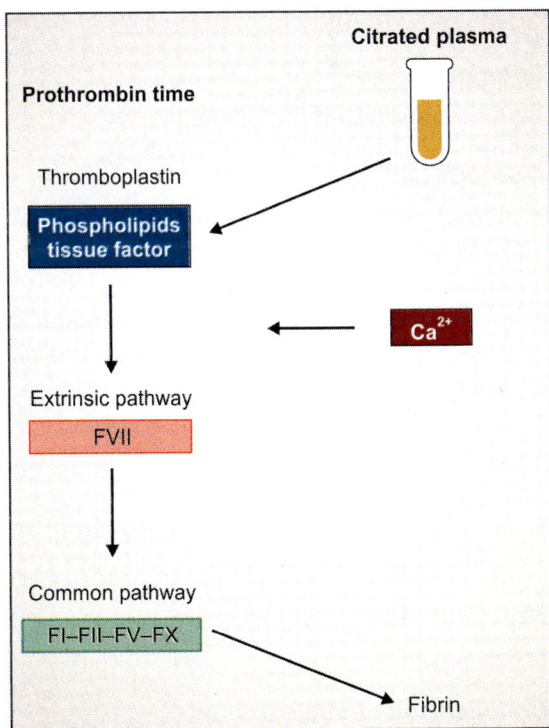

Fig. 2.1: Principle of prothrombin time

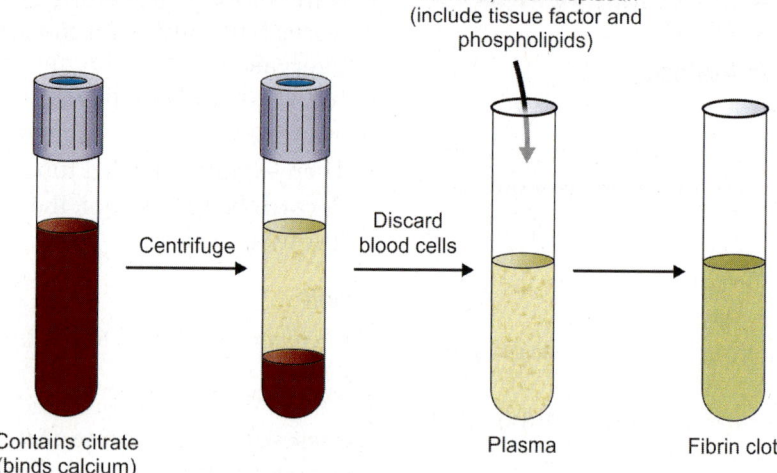

Fig. 2.2: Prothrombin time procedure

- Test tubes
- Stopwatch

Reagents
- Thromboplastin reagent contains tissue factor
- Calcium chloride

Specimen
Platelet poor citrated plasma.

Methods (Fig. 2.2)
- Anticoagulated blood is centrifuged at 3000–4000 revolutions per minute for 15–30 minutes.
- Plasma is separated and 0.1 ml is taken in glass test tube and is kept in water bath at 37°C.
- Add 0.1 ml of thromboplastin reagent and mix.
- After 1 minute, add 0.1 ml of calcium chloride solution.
- Start the stopwatch and record the time required for clot formation.

Normal Range
11–16 seconds

Prolongation of PT is seen in
- Patients taking oral anticoagulants

- Liver disease
- Vitamin K deficiency

4. ACTIVATED PARTIAL THROMBOPLASTIN TIME (APTT)
Assesses the coagulation factors in intrinsic pathway (factors XII, XI, IX, VIII) and common pathway (factors X, V, prothrombin and fibrinogen).

Principles (Fig. 2.3)
- Plasma is incubated with an activator, thus initiating the intrinsic pathway of coagulation
- Phospholipid and calcium are now added and time for clot formation is noted.

Reagents
- *Kaolin:* Contact activator
- Phospholipid
- Calcium chloride

Specimen
Platelet poor citrated plasma.

Methods (Fig. 2.4)
- Mix equal volumes of phospholipid reagent and calcium chloride solution in a test tube and keep in a water bath at 37°C.

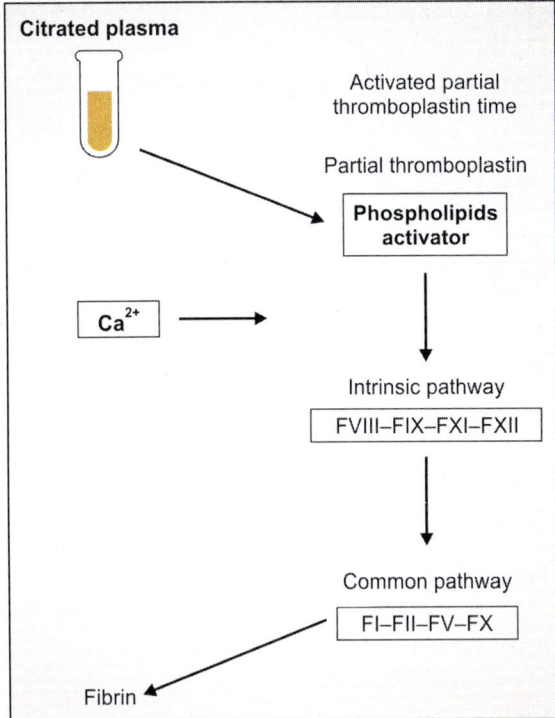

Fig. 2.3: Principle of APTT

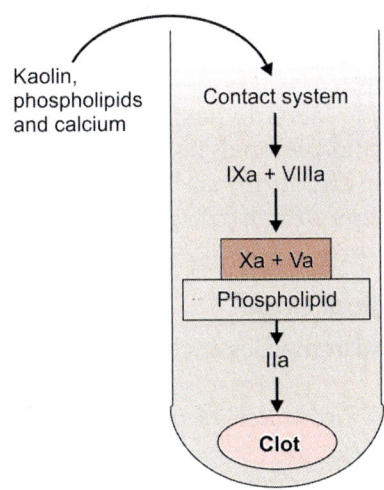

Fig. 2.4: APTT procedure

- Take 0.1 ml of platelet poor citrated plasma in another test tube and add 0.1 ml of kaolin solution.

- Incubate at 37°C in water bath for 10 minutes
- After 10 minutes, add 0.2 ml of phospholipid–calcium chloride mixture, and with the help of stopwatch, note the clotting time.

Normal Range

30–40 seconds

Prolonged APTT is seen in

- Hemophilia A or B
- Heparin therapy
- Liver disease
- Deficiencies of coagulation factors in intrinsic and common pathways.

5. THROMBIN TIME

Assesses the final step of coagulation, i.e. conversion of fibrinogen to fibrin by thrombin.

Principle

Thrombin is added to patients plasma and time required for clot formation is noted.

Reagent

Thrombin solution.

Specimen

Citrated platelet poor plasma.

Methods

- Take 0.1 ml of buffered saline in a test tube and add 0.1 ml of plasma.
- Clotting time is noted after addition of 0.1 ml of thrombin solution.

Normal Range

3 seconds.

Prolonged thrombin time is seen in

- *Disorders of fibrinogen:* Afibrinogenemia, hypofibrinogenemia, dysfibrinogenemia.
- Heparin therapy (heparin inhibits action of thrombin).

Automation in Hematology

What is Automation?

Automation is the process in which the computerized system has taken over the work performed by humans in laboratories.

INTRODUCTION

The hematological tests, which were performed by manual methods, had been replaced by machines.

At the peripheral centers, still manual methods are being used. Hematology analyzers, which generate the results at a fast rate and without errors, have widely replaced manual tests like WBC count, RBC count, platelet count, PCV, ESR, etc.

How is Automation Useful?

- Test reports can be obtained at a fast rate
- Large number of samples can run simultaneously
- Multiple tests can be interpreted with a single sample
- High accuracy of these test results as compared to tests performed manually
- Reduction in manpower
- Reducing the operator exposure to potential hazardous biological material.

Disadvantages of Automation

- Flagged reports (which require slide examination for confirmation)
- Expensive with high running costs
- Interfering factors for various test results.

Three stages of laboratory testing are
a. Pre-analytical
b. Analytical
c. Post-analytical

a. Pre-analytical Stage

- Concerned with sample or specimen processing
- Printed bar code labels are used for sample labeling
- Bar code labeling has reduced processing times and pre-analytical errors.
- Proper attention has been attributed for the steps of centrifugation, decapping, aliquoting, recapping, storage and retrieval.

b. Analytical Stage

Tasks and remedies included in this phase include:

1. *Sample introduction into the automation machine*
- Sample being taken up by the sample probe from the vaccutainer.
- Sample probes have a clot detection property, as clot can result in malfunction of the automated analyzer.
- Carry over contamination with one sample from another can be avoided by usage of wash solution in-between each pipetting.

2. Reagents

- Automated systems are classified as open reagent systems and close reagent systems.
- Open reagent system is one, in which reagents other than the instrument manufacture's reagents can be used and these systems are more flexible.
- Closed reagent system is one, in which only instrument manufacture's reagents can be used and is a more expensive system.
- For an individual test, a fixed proportion of sample volume and reagent volume should be used.

3. Incubation

- A proper temperature should be maintained in a system for proper test results.
- This can be achieved with the help of heat pumps or thermal rings inside the machine.

4. Detection

- Absorption spectroscopy is used in automated analyzers.
- Principle used in automation system for detection is electrochemiluminescence

c. Post-analytical Stage

- After a test sample is run, the electrical signals from the detector are interpreted by the computers as a digital signal.
- Multiple signals are interpreted and the results are displayed both as data and figures.

Parameters Measured by Hematology Analyzers

- RBC count
- Hemoglobin
- Mean cell volume
- Mean cell hemoglobin
- Mean cell hemoglobin concentration
- WBC count
- WBC differential
- Platelet count
- Red cell distribution width
- Reticulocyte count
- Mean platelet volume
- Platelet distribution width

Bone Marrow Examination

Bone marrow is the site of hematopoiesis in postnatal life.

During **infancy and early childhood**, hematopoiesis is seen all bones of the body.

Ribs, sternum, iliac bones, vertebrae, proximal end of long bones are the major sites of hematopoiesis in **late childhood.**

Sites of Bone Marrow Aspiration

Iliac crest, sternum, tibia, spinous processes of lumbar vertebrae.

In *bone marrow aspiration:* Bone marrow fluid is aspirated and smears are prepared on glass slides.

In *bone marrow biopsy (trephine biopsy):* Tissue of bone marrow is removed and processed in histopathology laboratory.

Indications for Bone Marrow Aspiration

- Unexplained cytopenias
- Suspected acute leukemia for classification and categorization.
- Suspected chronic myeloproliferative disorders.
- Suspected myelodyspalstic syndromes
- Metastatic tumors to the marrow
- Investigation of pyrexia of unknown origin
- Suspected storage disorder like Gaucher's disease or Niemann-Pick disease.
- Suspected infections like kala-azar, miliary tuberculosis, or histoplasmosis.

Indications for Bone Marrow Biopsy

- Dry tap as seen in myelofibrosis or leukemia
- Suspected aplastic anemia
- Suspected myelofibrosis
- Suspected hairy cell leukemia
- Staging of lymphoma

Processing of Marrow Specimens

1. *Bone marrow aspiration*
- Drop of a sample is placed on a slide
- Smears are prepared by a spreader
- Marrow particles are carried behind the spreader and cellular trails are produced while spreading.
- Smears are dried and stained with Romanowsky stains.

2. *Bone marrow trephine biopsy*
- Biopsy specimen is fixed with 10% formalin
- Biopsy is processed to obtain paraffin wax blocks.
- 4 microns thick sections, 5 in number are cut in a stepwise fashion.
- These sections are stained with hematoxylin and eosin.
- Prussian blue, Giemsa stain will be helpful in diagnosis.

Information Obtained from Bone Marrow Aspiration

1. Morphology
2. Cytochemistry
3. Iron stain
4. Immunophenotyping
5. Culture

Studies which can be done on bone marrow aspirate smears

- Romanowsky stain
- Iron stain
- Cytochemistry
- Molecular genetics
- Immunophenotying
- Culture

Information received from bone marrow biopsy

1. Cellularity (normocellular, hypercellular or hypocellular)
2. Architecture (well preserved or poorly preserved)
3. Fibrosis (present or absent)
4. Focal lesions (present or absent)
5. Bone structure (preserved or lost)

Studies which can be done on bone marrow biopsy

- Hematoxylin and eosin stain
- Reticulin stain
- Immunohistochemistry

Cellular Components in Blood Film

Peripheral blood smear is examined for

a. Red blood cells morphology
b. *White blood cells:* Differential count
c. Platelet count
d. *Parasites:* Malaria, filaria

Peripheral blood smear comprises three parts: Head, body and tail.

1. Red Blood Cells (RBCs)

- Examined at the tail end of smear
- Normal red cells are 7–8 microns in size with an area of central pallor.
- Size of normal red cell corresponds to the size of the nucleus of a small lymphocyte.

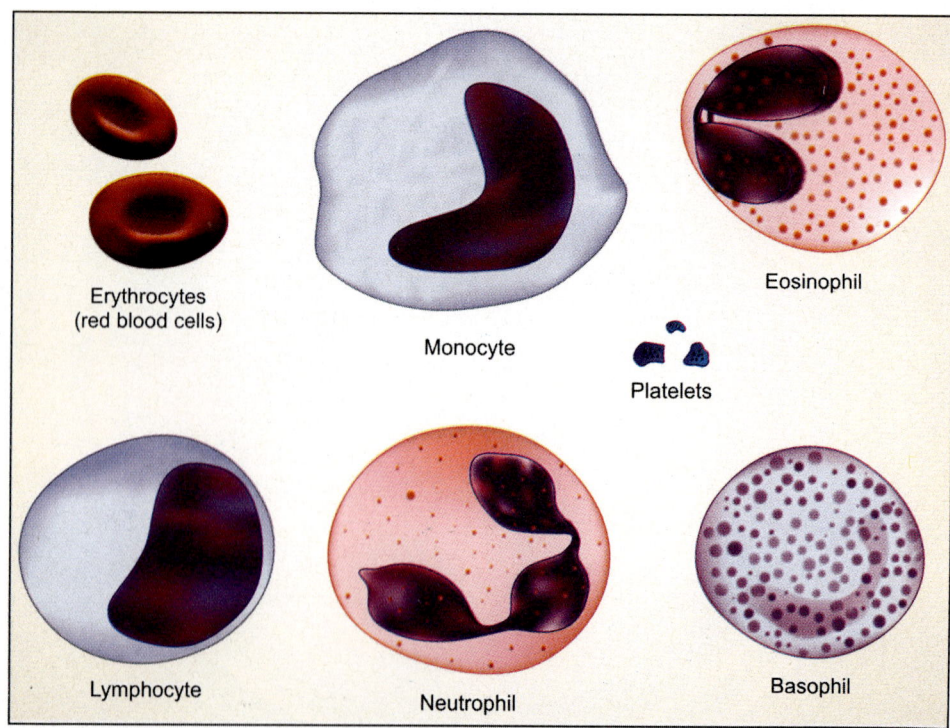

Fig. 5.1: Types of blood cells

- In normal blood smear, RBCs appear normocytic normochromic.
- RBCs smaller than normal are called microcytes.
- RBCs larger than normal are called macrocytes.
- RBCs which are large and oval in shape are called macro-ovalocytes.

2. White Blood Cells (WBCs)

Differential leukocyte count (DLC) comprises neutrophils, lymphocytes, eosinophils, basophils and monocytes (Fig. 5.1).

a. Polymorphonuclear neutrophils
- Neutrophil measures 14–15 microns in size
- Cytoplasm contains granules
- Nucleus has 2–5 lobes
- Normal count is 40–75%

b. Eosinophils
- Measures 15–16 microns
- Bilobed nucleus and cytoplasm have large orange-red granules
- Normal count is 1–6%

c. Basophils
- Measures 9–12 microns
- Cytoplasm contains large, coarse, purple granules
- Normal count is 0–1%

d. Monocytes
- Largest leukocytes
- Measures 15–20 microns
- Cells have abundant cytoplasm and irregular shape oval or clefted nucleus.
- Normal count is 2–10%

e. Lymphocytes
- Two types of lymphocytes—small and large
- Small lymphocytes are 7–8 microns in size, with blue cytoplasm.
- Large lymphocytes are 10–15 microns in size, with pale blue cytoplasm.
- Normal count is 20–40%.

3. Platelets

Small, 1–3 microns in diameter, purple structures.

Coagulation Cascade

A. In laboratory (Fig. 6.1)
Intrinsic pathway: Clotting is initiated by phospholipids, calcium, and negatively charged substance such as glass beads.

Extrinsic pathway: Clotting is initiated with source of tissue factor.

B. In blood vessel: Tissue factor is the major initiator of coagulation.

Assessment of coagulation pathway is done by
a. *Prothrombin time (PT) assay:* Assesses the function of proteins in the extrinsic pathway (factors VII, X, V, II, and fibrinogen)
b. *Partial thromboplastin time (PTT) assay:* Assesses the function of the proteins in the intrinsic pathway (factors XII, XI, IX, VIII, X, V, II, and fibrinogen)

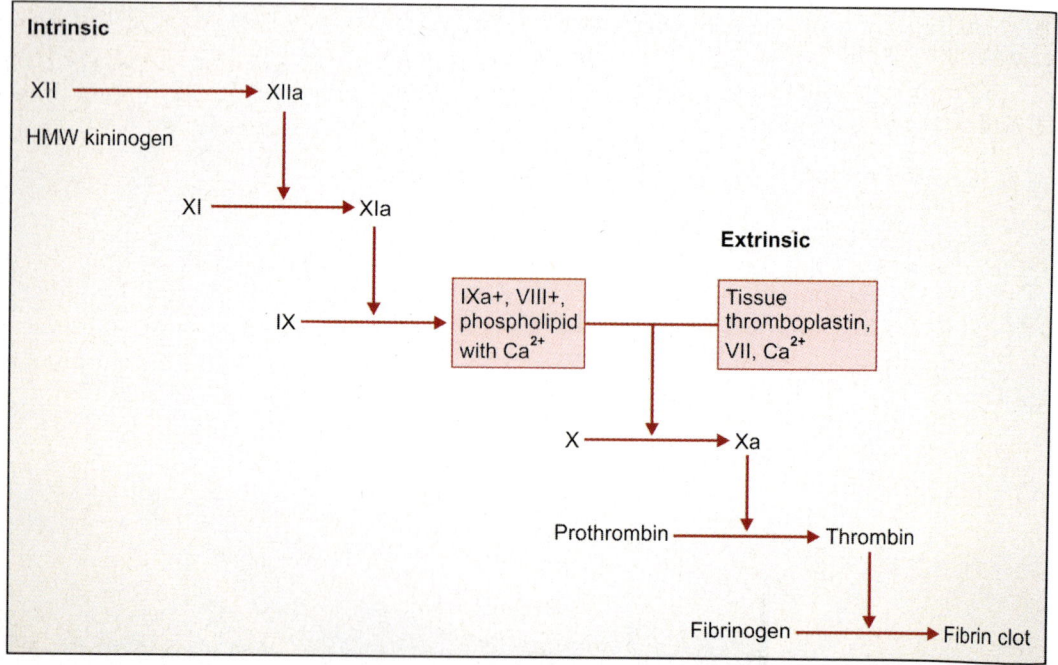

Fig. 6.1: Coagulation cascade

COAGULATION DISORDERS

A. Inherited Disorders

Hemophilia A (Factor VIII Deficiency)

- Most common hereditary disease associated with life-threatening bleeding, caused by mutations in factor VIII.
- Patient presents with spontaneous hemorrhages into joints (hemarthrosis).
- Patients have prolonged PTT and a normal PT.

Hemophilia B (Christmas Disease, Factor IX Deficiency)

- Factors VIII and IX function together to activate factor X.
- PTT is prolonged and the PT is normal.

B. Acquired Disorders

Vitamin K deficiency and liver disorders result in the impaired synthesis of factors II, VII, IX, X and protein C.

ANTICOAGULANTS

- Laboratory instruments, blood transfusion bags, medical and surgical pieces of equipment will become non-functional, if the anticoagulant is not used as the blood will clot inside them.
- These anticoagulants inhibit calcium ions and thus inhibit the coagulant cascade.

Examples
- EDTA (ethylenediaminetetra-acetic acid) binds and chelates calcium
- Sodium citrate
- Oxalate

Citrate containing anticoagulants: Acid citrate dextrose, citrate phosphate dextrose, sodium citrate, citrate phosphate dextrose with adenine (CPD-A), Alsever's solution.

Anticoagulants used according to the vacutainer used
- *Blue vacutainer (used for coagulation studies):* 3.2% trisodium citrate (2.7 ml of blood + 0.3 ml of anticoagulant = 9:1)
- *Lavender (for routine hematological investigations):* Dipotassium EDTA
- *Grey (for blood glucose):* Dipotassium EDTA contains sodium fluoride (antimetabolite)
- *Black (for ESR):* 3.8% trisodium citrate (1.6 ml of blood and 0.4 ml of citrate = 4:1)
- *Red (for serum studies):* Without anticoagulant (4 ml of blood is collected)
- *Green* for enzyme studies, osmotic fragility test, arterial blood gas analysis contains lithium heparin.

Composition and Functions of Blood

1. COMPOSITION OF BLOOD

Blood is made up of plasma, RBCs, WBCs and platelets.

a. *Plasma*
   - Straw-colored fluid
   - 90% is water and also contains electrolytes such as sodium, potassium and proteins.

b. *RBCs*
   - Main function of RBCs is to carry oxygen.
   - RBC has a lifespan of 120 days, before it is broken down in spleen.

c. *WBCs:* Composed of neutrophils, lymphocytes, monocytes, eosinophils and platelets.

d. *Platelets:* Disc-shaped fragments involved in clotting of blood.

2. FUNCTIONS OF BLOOD

a. *Transportation*
   - Blood carries gases (CO_2, O_2) between the lungs and rest of the body.
   - Nutrients from the digestive tract from site of absorption to the body.
   - Waste products to be detoxified by the liver or kidneys.
   - Hormones from the glands in which they are produced to their target cells.
   - Provides heat and warmth to the skin to regulate the body temperature.

b. *Maintaining hemostasis*

c. *Protection:* Blood plays a role in inflammation.
   - WBCs destroy the cancer cells
   - Antibodies destroy the pathogens
   - Platelets initiate the clotting and help in minimizing the blood loss.

d. *Regulation: Blood helps regulate*
   - pH by interaction between acids and bases.
   - Water balance by transferring water to and from the tissues.

Coombs' Test
(Anti-globin Test)

Two types

a. Direct antiglobulin test

b. Indirect antiglobulin test

a. Direct Antiglobulin (Coombs') Test (DAT)
(Fig. 8.1)

- Detects antibodies or complement or both attached to the red cells.
- Principle: Red cells of the patient are washed with normal saline (to remove unbound antibodies) and anti-human globulin (AHG) reagent is added.
- Agglutination of red cells indicates positive test.

Causes of positive test: Autoimmune hemolytic anemia, hemolytic diseases of newborn, hemolytic transfusion reaction, drug-induced hemolysis.

b. Indirect Antiglobulin (Coombs') Test (IAT)
(Fig. 8.2)

- Detects the presence of antibodies in the serum, directed against the red cell antigens.
- Patient's serum is incubated with red cells (donor or screening) to allow binding of antibodies in serum to red cell antigens.
- After washing of red cells in saline (to remove unbound antibodies), anti-human globulin reagent is added.
- Agglutination of the red cells denotes positive test.

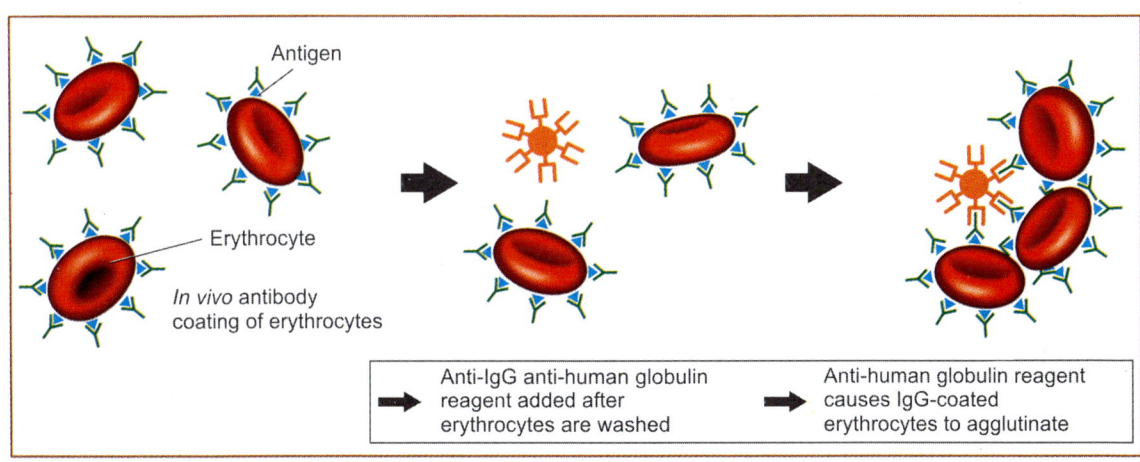

Antigen

Erythrocyte

In vivo antibody coating of erythrocytes

| Anti-IgG anti-human globulin reagent added after erythrocytes are washed | Anti-human globulin reagent causes IgG-coated erythrocytes to agglutinate |

Fig. 8.1: Direct Coombs' test

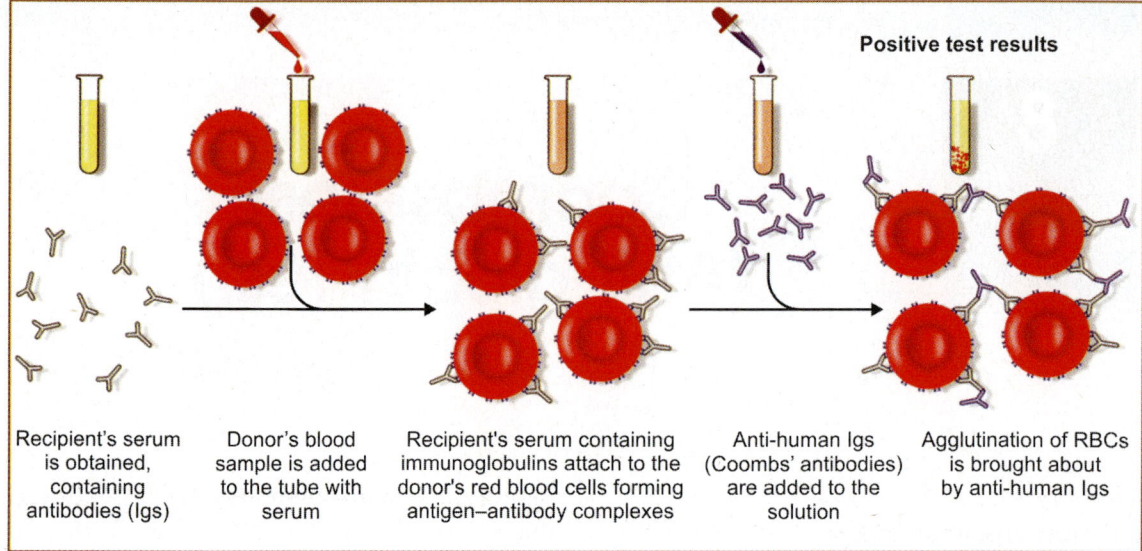

Positive test results

| Recipient's serum is obtained, containing antibodies (Igs) | Donor's blood sample is added to the tube with serum | Recipient's serum containing immunoglobulins attach to the donor's red blood cells forming antigen–antibody complexes | Anti-human Igs (Coombs' antibodies) are added to the solution | Agglutination of RBCs is brought about by anti-human Igs |

Fig. 8.2: Indirect Coombs' test

Uses of indirect agglutination test
- Cross-matching before transfusion
- Antibody screening and identification
- For detecting anti-Rh antibodies in the serum.

Erythropoiesis

Stages of Erythropoiesis (Fig. 9.1)

1. *Pro-erythroblast:* Large cell, open chromatin, with blue cytoplasm.
2. *Basophilic (early) erythroblast:* Fine nuclear clumped chromatin.
3. *Intermediate erythroblast (polychromato-philic):* Smaller cell with coarse clumped chromatin.
4. *Late erythroblast (orthochromatic):* Small, dense, pyknotic and eccentric nucleus
5. *Reticulocyte (polychromatic RBC):* No nucleus and blue-gray color cytoplasm.
6. *Erythrocytes:* No nucleus and red cytoplasm.

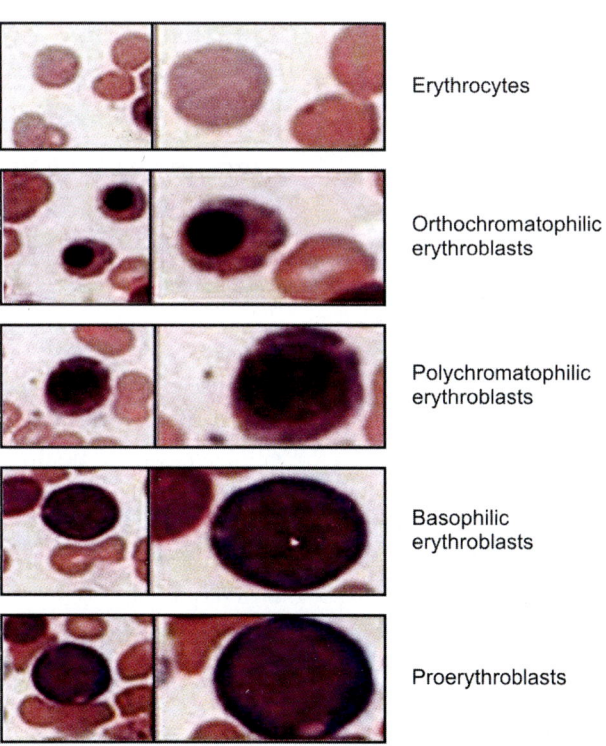

Erythrocytes

Orthochromatophilic erythroblasts

Polychromatophilic erythroblasts

Basophilic erythroblasts

Proerythroblasts

Fig. 9.1: Stages of erythropoiesis

10

Erythrocyte Sedimentation Rate (ESR)

- ESR measures the rate of sedimentation (settling) of erythrocytes in the anti-coagulated whole blood.
- Anticoagulated blood sample is allowed to stand in a glass tube for 1 hour.

Stages of ESR

Three stages:

- *Stage 1: Formation of Rouleaux (10 minutes):* Red cells stack together like a pack of coins
- *Stage 2: Sinking of Rouleaux (40 minutes):* Rapid and constant sedimentation.
- *Stage 3: Packing of Rouleaux (10 minutes):* Slow sedimentation.

Why is ESR Measured?

- Measurement is indicated in cases of infections, inflammatory disorders or cancers.
- To monitor the disease activity in tuberculosis, arthritis.

Methods of Estimation of ESR

- Westergren method
- Wintrobe method
- Zeta sedimentation ratio
- Micro-ESR.

Westergren Method

Equipment and reagents:
1. *Westergren's ESR tube* (Fig. 10.1)

- Straight glass pipette measuring 300 mm in length
- Calibrated in mm from 0 to 200 (top to bottom)
- Internal diameter is around 2.5 mm
- Tube should be dry and clean

2. *Westergren stand:* Holds the tube in a motionless, vertical position.

3. *Anticoagulant diluted solution:* Tri-sodium citrate dehydrate is the anticoagulant of choice.

Specimen Collection

Venous blood is collected in trisodium citrate solution in the ratio of 4:1 (blood:citrate).

Methods

- Mix anticoagulated blood thoroughly
- Westergren tube is filled with the blood sample up to the zero mark.
- There should be no air bubbles while filling the tube.
- Tube is placed in a vertical position in ESR stand and is left undisturbed for 1 hour.
- After 1 hour, read the height of the column of plasma above the red cell column in mm.

Result

Express the result as erythrocyte sedimentation rate = ... mm in 1 hour.

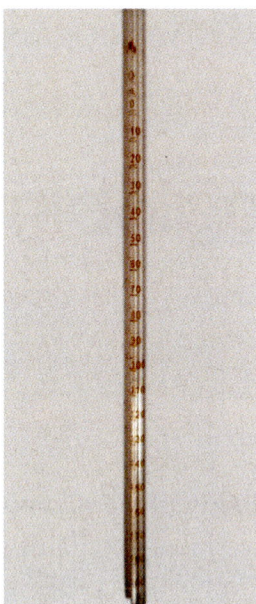

Fig. 10.1: Westergren's tube

Following points should be taken care of
- Test should be performed at room temperature
- Use the correct proportion of blood and anticoagulant
- ESR tube should be in a vertical position.

Normal Values
- Males <50 years: 0–15 mm in 1 hour
- Females <50 years: 0–20 mm in 1 hour
- Children: 0–10 mm in 1 hour.

Hemoglobin Estimation

INDICATIONS FOR HEMOGLOBIN ESTIMATION

- To determine the presence and severity of anemia: Anemia refers to low hemoglobin levels.
- To diagnose polycythemia, i.e. increased hemoglobin levels.
- To monitor the response of treatment in patients with anemia.
- To estimate red cell indices.

METHODS OF ESTIMATION OF HEMOGLOBIN

- Calorimetric method:
    - Sahli's acid hematin method
    - Cyanmethemoglobin method
- Gasometric method
- Chemical methods
- Specific gravity method.

a. Sahli's Acid Hematin Method

Principles

- Blood is mixed with acid solution, which coverts hemoglobin into brown-colored acid hematin.
- This solution is diluted with water till the brown color matches that of brown glass standard.
- Hemoglobin value is read directly from the scale.

Equipment

- Sahli's hemoglobinometer consists of Sahli's hemoglobin tube (marked in gm%) and a comparator with a brown glass standard.
- Sahli's pipette or hemoglobin pipette (marked as 20 microliter or 0.02 ml).
- Stirrer
- Pipette

Reagents

- N/10 hydrochloric acid
- Distilled water

Specimen

EDTA blood

Methods

- Put N/10 HCl into Sahli's graduated hemoglobin tube up to the mark of 2 gm
- Take the blood sample in Sahli's pipette up to 20 microliters mark.
- Add blood sample to the acid solution
- Mix with a glass stirrer
- Allow it to stand for 10 minutes
- Add distilled water drop by drop till the color of the solution matches that of brown glass standard.
- Take the reading of the lower meniscus from the tube in grams.

Disadvantages of Sahli's Method

- For maximum development of color of acid hematin, it takes an hour, however, 95% of the color is attained in 10 minutes and the reading in our test is taken at the end of ten minutes.
- HbF seen in infants will not be converted to acid hematin on treatment with HCl, hence this method is not used for detecting hemoglobin of infants.
- Matching color with brown glass can give false interpretation of the results and hence false values.

b. Cyanmethemoglobin Method

Method of choice for estimation of hemoglobin as all forms of hemoglobin are converted to cyanmethemoglobin.

Reagents

1. *Drabkin's solution*
   - Potassium ferricyanide—200 mg
   - Potassium cyanide—50 mg
   - Potassium dihydrogen phosphate—140 mg
   - Non-ionic detergent—1 ml
   - Distilled water to make 1000 ml
2. Cyanmethemoglobin standard solution with known hemoglobin value.

Principles

- Blood is mixed with Drabkin's solution
- Erythrocytes are lysed producing hemoglobin.
- Potassium ferricyanide converts hemoglobin to methemoglobin, which combines with potassium cyanide to form cyanmethemoglobin.

- Absorbance of the solution is measured in a spectrophotometer at 540 nm wavelength.
- To know the amount of hemoglobin in unknown sample, its absorbance is compared with standard cyanmethemoglobin solution.

Equipment

1. Photoelectric calorimeter or spectrophotometer
2. Sahli's pipette marked at 20 cu mm
3. Pipette 5 ml

Specimen

EDTA blood

Methods

- In a test tube, take 5 ml of Drabkin's solution and add 20 cu mm of blood (dilution factor of 1:251).
- Mix the solution by inverting several times and allow it to stand for 5 minutes.
- Transfer the test sample to a cuvette and read the absorbance in a spectrophotometer at 540 nm.
- Also note the absorption of standard solution, which is read against a reagent blank (i.e. Drabkin's solution)

Hemoglobin in gm/dl =

$$\frac{\text{Absorbance of test sample}}{\text{Absorbance of the standard}} \times \frac{\text{Concentration of standard}}{100} \times \text{Dilution factor}$$

Hemoglobin and its Variants

- Hemoglobin is made up of heme and globin
- Globin protein is composed of different types of chains, named alpha, beta, delta and gamma.

Normal hemoglobin types include

a. *Hemoglobin A:* Makes up 95–98% of hemoglobin in adults, contains two alpha (α) and two beta (β) protein chains.

b. *Hemoglobin A_2:* Makes up 2–3% of hemoglobin found in adults, contains two alpha (α) and two delta (δ) protein chains.

c. *Hemoglobin F:* Makes up 1–2% of hemoglobin, found in adults, contains two alpha (α) and two gamma (γ) protein chains.

Hemoglobin Variants

- Globin gene mutation, results in structurally altered hemoglobin like HbS (sickle cell anemia).
- Globin gene mutation, results in altered hemoglobin production as seen in thalassemia.
- HbE disease and HbE trait
- HbC disease and HbC trait
- *Hemoglobin F (HbF):* Elevated levels are seen in beta-thalassemia, sickle cell anemia, or in hereditary persistence of fetal hemoglobin.
- *Hemoglobin H (HbH):* Seen in patients of alpha-thalassemia, and are composed of four beta (β) globin chains, produced due to shortage of alpha (α) chains.
- *Hemoglobin Bart:* Seen in patients of alpha-thalassemia, and are composed of four gamma (γ) chains, produced due to shortage of alpha (α) chains.
- *Hemoglobin SC disease:* Inheritance of one beta S gene and one beta C gene.
- *Sickle cell—hemoglobin D disease:* Inheritance of one hemoglobin S gene and one hemoglobin D—Los Angeles (or D-Punjab) gene.
- *Hemoglobin E—beta-thalassemia disease:* Individuals are heterozygous for hemoglobin E gene and beta-thalassemia gene.

Thalassemia
Clinical Course

- Due to deficient hemoglobin chain synthesis, there occurs diminished survival of RBCs.
- Also these, unpaired alpha chains in alpha-thalassemia and beta chains in beta-thalassemia form RBC inclusions.
- Inclusions lead to membrane damage, which result in RBC destruction.
- Due to anemia, patient requires frequent blood transfusions.
- Children, who are not treated with blood transfusion, die at an early age.
- Frequent blood transfusion results in iron overload in patients blood and in their organs.

- Cardiac disease is an important cause of death, due to progressive iron overload.
- Hematopoietic stem cell transplantation can offer cure.

Diagnosis

Peripheral Smear

- Microcytic hypochromic anemia
- Marked variation in size (anisocytosis) and shape (poikilocytosis) of RBCs
- Target cells (hemoglobin collects in the center of the cell), basophilic stippling, and fragmented red cells are seen.

Levels of normal hemoglobin components and its variants in different disorders

- HbA_2 is elevated (4–8%) in beta-thalassemia trait
- HbF will be elevated in thalassemia
- HbA will be reduced in thalassemia
- HbS will be seen in sickle cell anemia.

HEMOGLOBIN ELECTROPHORESIS

Electrophoresis is the movement of hemoglobin proteins in an electric field at a fixed pH.

Principle

An electric field is applied through a supporting medium and the solutes migrate in that field, according to their net charge.

Example

For thalassemia, alkaline electrophoresis is performed.

Principles of Hemoglobin Electrophoresis
(Fig. 12.1)

- It is performed to find out abnormal forms of hemoglobin (hemoglobinopathy).
- Different types of hemoglobin separated include HbA, HbA_2, HbF, HbS, HbC.
- Tissue extracts are introduced into the sample wells in gel.
- An electrical field is applied, and proteins with net negative charge will migrate towards the cathode end of the field.

Cellulose Acetate Method at Alkaline pH

Principles

- In an alkaline pH (8.2–8.6), hemoglobin is negatively charged molecule and migrate towards the cathode.
- Various hemoglobin molecules move at different rates depending on their net negative charge, which in turn is controlled by the composition (amino acids) of the Hb molecule (globin chain).
- One end of cellulose acetate strip is immersed in the buffer (pH 8.2–8.6) on the cathode side and the other end is placed in the buffer on the anode side.
- An electric current of specific voltage is allowed to run.
- During electrophoresis, hemoglobin molecules migrate toward the cathode because of their negative charge.
- Cellulose acetate membrane is then stained in order to color the proteins (hemoglobin).
- By noting the distance, each hemoglobin has migrated, and comparing this distance with

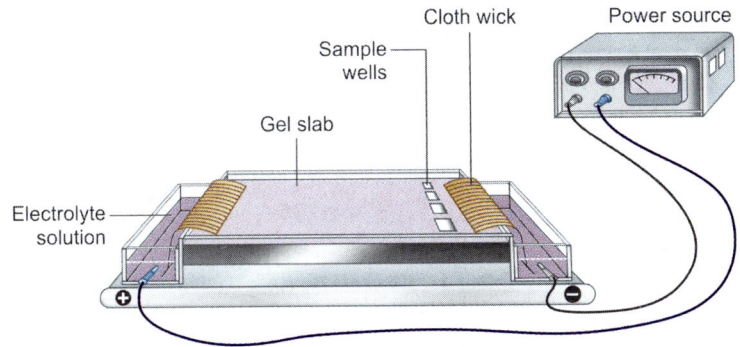

Fig. 12.1: Principle of electrophoresis

the migration distance of known controls, the types of hemoglobin may be identified.

Migration of Hemoglobin in Electrophoresis
(Fig. 12.2)

- Of the normal hemoglobin in an adult, HbA is the fastest, followed by HbF

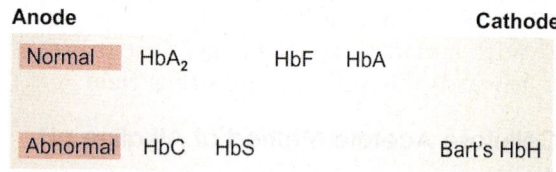

Fig. 12.2: Pattern of distribution of abnormal hemoglobin on electrophoresis

- HbA_2 moves only slightly from the point of origin near the anode.
- Abnormal hemoglobin shows the following migration patterns: HbC migrates with HbA_2 near the anode.
- HbS lies between hemoglobin A_2 and hemoglobin F.
- HbH and Bart are unstable and very fast moving, placing them past HbA.

Note: All hemoglobin specimens that show an abnormal electrophoresis pattern in alkaline media (cellulose acetate agar) should undergo electrophoresis on an acid citrate agar.

Hemostasis

Definition: Mechanism by which blood clots at the site of vascular injury.

Sequence of Events (Fig. 13.1)

a. *Arteriolar vasoconstriction:* Arteriole, where there occurs an injury, will undergo constriction.

b. *Primary hemostasis*
- Brought about by platelets
- Platelets adhere to the vessel wall and get activated.
- Activated platelets will release mediators and bring about platelet aggregation and formation of primary hemostatic plug.

c. *Secondary hemostasis*
- Tissue factor released at the endothelial cell injury site will result in activation of coagulation pathway.
- This activation of coagulation cascade results in formation of secondary hemostatic plug, due to deposition of fibrin.

d. *Clot stabilization:* Tissue plasminogen activator limits the clot size at the site of injury.

PLATELET DISORDERS

- Following vascular injury, platelets adhere to the vWF exposed due to endothelial cell damage.

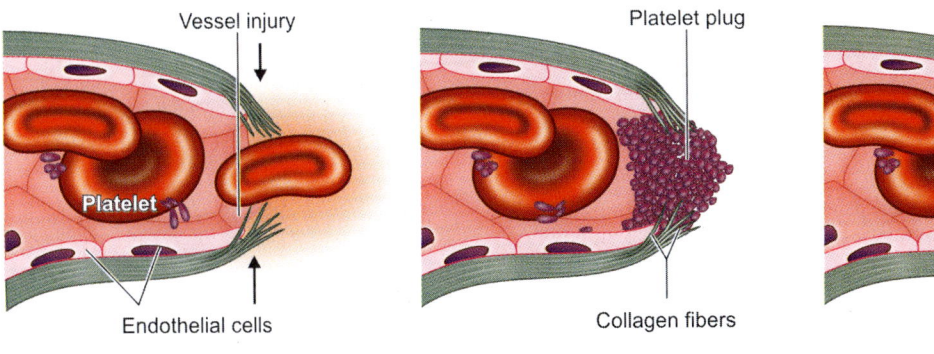

Vessel spasm   **Platelet plug formation**   **Blood clot**

Fig. 13.1: Formation of hemostatic plug

- Platelets adhere to vWF through platelet surface receptor glycoprotein (Gp)Ib-IXa.

von Willebrand Disease

- Occurs due to deficiency of vWF
- Most common inherited bleeding disorder of humans.
- Spontaneous bleeding from mucous membranes (e.g. epistaxis), excessive bleeding from wounds, or menorrhagia.

Bernard-Soulier Syndrome

- Occurs due to deficiency of GpIb-IXa, a receptor for vWF.
- GpIb-IXa is essential for normal platelet adhesion to the subendothelial extracellular matrix.

- Bleeding due to defective platelet adhesion to subendothelial matrix.

Activated platelets produce thromboxane A_2, which brings about platelet aggregation. Platelets have GpIIb-IIIa receptors on their surface, which increases their affinity for fibrinogen.

Glycoprotein IIb-IIIa leads to binding of fibrinogen and forms bridges among platelets, bringing about platelet aggregation.

Glanzmann Thrombasthenia

- Bleeding disorder due to inherited deficiency of GpIIb-IIIa, due to defective platelet aggregation.
- Glycoprotein IIb-IIIa (acts as a bridge between platelets by binding fibrinogen).

LE Cell

- LE cell is usually a neutrophil/polymorph that has ingested the altered nucleus of another polymorph.
- LE cell appears as basophilic, homogeneous mass that stains purplish brown.
- Lobes of the ingesting polymorph appear wrapped around the ingested material.
- Polymorphs can collect around an altered nuclear material and form a "rosette".

LE cells can be seen in
- Systemic lupus erythematosus
- Rheumatoid arthritis
- Discoid lupus erythematosus.

Methods of Demonstration of LE Cell

- Clotted blood
- Defibrinated blood
- Citrated or heparinized blood
- Rotary method.

The Rotary Method

1. 1 ml of patient's blood collected in heparin is transferred into a glass tube.
2. Four glass beads are added and the tube is sealed.
3. Preparation is rotated at 33 rpm at room temperature for 30 minutes and placed at 37°C for 10–15 minutes.
4. Contents of the tube are transferred to a Wintrobe tube and centrifuged for 10 minutes.
5. Buffy coat smears are prepared, dried in the air, fixed in methanol and are stained with Romanowsky stain.

Note
- Some degree of trauma to the leukocytes is necessary for a successful preparation of LE cell.
- As anti-nuclear antibodies do not act upon healthy living leukocytes.
- A good method of achieving the necessary degree of trauma is to rotate the whole blood sample to which glass beads have been added.

Interpretation (Fig. 14.1)

- LE cells are seen at the edge of a smear
- 500 polymorphs are counted before a negative result is given.
- *Note:* LE cells must be differentiated from "tart cells" which are usually monocytes that have phagocytosed the nucleus of a lymphocyte.

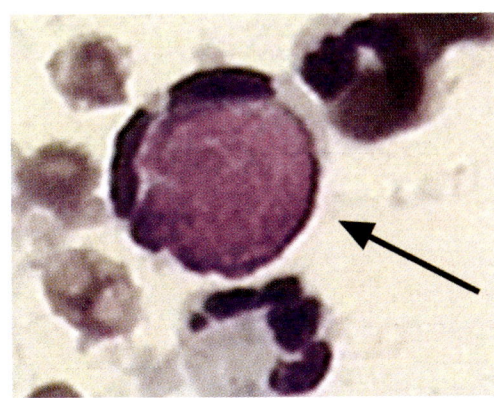

Fig. 14.1: LE cell (arrow)

Leukopoiesis

Definition: Process of generating white blood cells (leucocyte) from pluripotent hematopoietic stem cells of bone marrow.

There are two significant pathways:

a. *Myelopoiesis* in which leukocytes in blood are derived from myeloid stem cells.

b. *Lymphopoiesis* in which leukocytes of the lymphatic system (lymphocytes) are generated from the lymphoid stem cells.

- From the early progenitor cell with lymphoid potential, there arises pro-NK cell, pro-B cell and pro-T cell which give rise to NK cell, B cell and T cell , respectively.

- From CFU-mix (colony forming unit-mix population) arises myeloblast, monoblast, eosinophiloblast which give rise to neutrophils, monocyte, and eosinophil, respectively

- From CFU-b/M/E arises basophiloblast, megakaryoblast and erythroblast which give rise to basophils, platelets and erythrocytes, respectively.

Leukemia

Leukemia is defined as cancer of blood cells.

- Bone marrow normally produces hematopoietic elements in mature form into the peripheral blood.

- When bone marrow produces increased number of precursor cells, there occurs an increase number of precursor cells in the blood too.

- As the blood cells are divided into myeloid and lymphoid precursors, there occurs myeloid and lymphoid leukemia.

- To be precise, precursors are further classified into varying populations.

Note: To learn more about the hematopoietic cell lines, kindly see chapter on leukopoiesis.

- Out of these precursor cell populations, if there occurs increase in number of blasts which make up more than 20% of the myeloid or lymphoid lineage cells, only than the term leukemia is used.

- So, in simple terms, if there are more than 20% of lymphoblasts in the bone marrow or peripheral blood, we report it as acute lymphoblastic leukemia (ALL).

- And, if there occurs more than 20% of myeloblasts in the bone marrow or peripheral blood, we report it as acute myeloid leukemia (AML).

- Leukemia can also be chronic and can involve both lymphoid and myeloid series of cells and are termed, respectively, as chronic lymphocytic leukemia (CLL) and chronic myeloid leukemia (CML).

- In CLL, there occurs increase proliferation of abnormal lymphoid cells.

- In CML, there occurs an increase in proliferation of precursors of myeloid lineage cells and the blast population remains less than 20%.

What is Responsible for Production of Abnormal Immature Cells?

- Due to genetic mutations in chromosomes of these patients, there occurs abnormal cell proliferation in the bone marrow.

- Ionizing radiation for treatment of tumors

- Accidental exposure of ionizing radiation can result in abnormal cellular proliferation in marrow

- Viruses, dyes and drugs are other responsible agents.

Clinical Features

- Patient presents with enlargement of lymph nodes, spleen, and liver.

- As the bone marrow function is not proper, hence there can be associated anemia, leukopenia and thrombocytopenia (i.e. pancytopenia).

- Because of these abnormalities in the normal cell production, these patients are predisposed for infections, fever, bleeding tendency and symptoms related to anemia.
- If leukemic cells spread to CSF, testes, brain, it is associated with poor prognosis.

Treatment

- For remission, different chemotherapeutic regimens are used, but invariably patients come back with the disease again after a gap of few months to years (called relapse).
- Bone marrow transplantation has shown promising results for curing these patients.

Osmotic Fragility Test

- Red cells are suspended in decreasing concentrations of hypotonic saline, to determine the ability of RBCs to withstand osmotic stress.
- In hypotonic solutions, water enters red cells causing cellular swelling, followed by RBC lysis.
- Normal RBCs are biconcave and disc shaped, have high surface area to volume ratio and therefore can increase their volume up to 70% before they are lysed.
- With normal RBCs hemolysis starts at saline concentration of 0.5 gm/dl and is complete at 0.30 gm/dl.
- In contrast, spherocytes have decreased surface area to volume ratio, and can undergo lysis earlier than normal RBCs.
- In presence of spherocytes, red cells show beginning of hemolysis at 0.6 to 0.8 gm/dl, i.e. increased osmotic fragility.
- Osmotic fragility is decreased in thalassemia, due to presence of target cells, since target cells have increased surface volume.
- Sensitivity of the test can be increased by incubating the red cells at 37°C for 24 hours before performing the test (osmotic fragility test after incubation).

Procedure

1. Make a stock solution (A) of 10 gm/L
   - NaCl—90 gm

- Na_2HPO_4—13.6 gm
- NaH_2PO_4—2.4 gm
- Distilled water—1000 ml

2. *Working solution:* Prepare 1 gm/dl buffered sodium chloride (NaCl) solution by mixing 10 ml of solution A and 90 ml of distilled water.

3. Prepare working solutions in centrifuge tubes as follows (Figs 17.1 and 17.2):

S.no. of test tube	NaCl concen- tration	NaCl	Distilled water	Blood (sample)
1.	100%	5.0 ml	X	0.05 ml
2.	90%	4.5 ml	0.5 ml	0.05 ml
3.	75%	3.75 ml	1.25 ml	0.05 ml
4.	65%	3.25 ml	1.75 ml	0.05 ml
5.	60%	3.00 ml	2.00 ml	0.05 ml
6.	55%	2.75 ml	2.25 ml	0.05 ml
7.	50%	2.50 ml	2.50 ml	0.05 ml
8.	45%	2.25 ml	2.75 ml	0.05 ml
9.	35%	1.75 ml	3.25 ml	0.05 ml
10.	30%	1.50 ml	3.50 ml	0.05 ml
11.	20%	1.00 ml	4.00 ml	0.05 ml
12.	10%	0.50 ml	4.50 ml	0.05 ml
13.	0	0.00 ml	5.00 ml	0.05 ml

- Mix well. Keep at room temperature for 30 minutes, centrifuge.
- Read the results in a spectrometer at a wavelength of 540 nm.

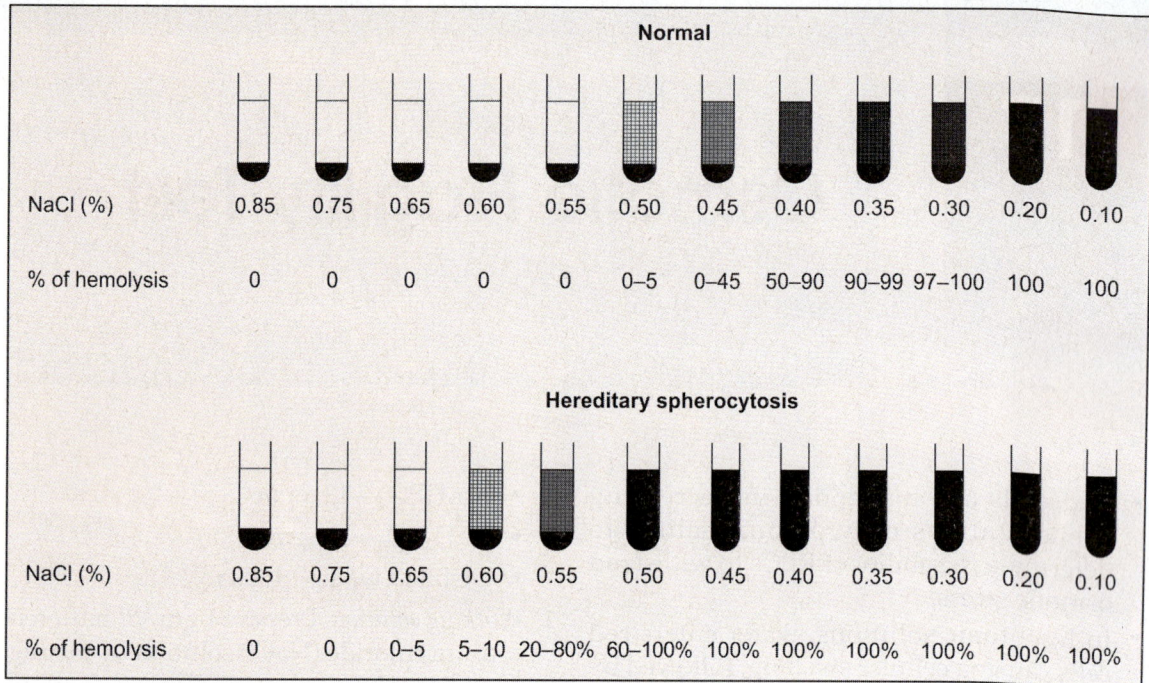

Fig. 17.1: Osmotic fragility is increased in hereditary spherocytosis as the hemolysis starts at lower concentration gradients of sodium chloride

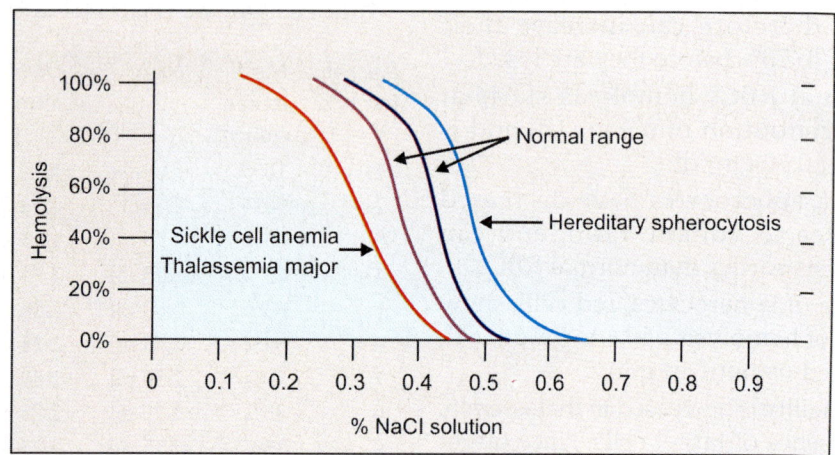

Fig. 17.2: Left shift to the normal range (reduced OF) is seen in sickle cell anemia and thalassemia. Right shift (increased OF) is seen in hereditary spherocytosis

Calculation

$$\% \text{ of hemolysis} = \frac{\text{Optical density of the sample}}{\text{Optical density of tube (showing complete hemolysis)}} \times 100$$

Packed Cell Volume (PCV)

- Volume occupied by RBCs when a sample of anticoagulated blood is centrifuged
- Also called hematocrit.

Uses of PCV

- Detection of the presence or absence of anemia or polycythemia.
- Estimation of red cell indices
- Estimation of hemoglobin using a simple calculation

  PCV = Hemoglobin multiplied by (×) 3

  For example: If hemoglobin is 15 gm%, than PCV will be 45%.

Methods of Estimation

1. Wintrobe method
2. Microhematocrit method.

1. Wintrobe Method

Equipment

a. Wintrobe tube (Fig. 18.1):
- Tube is 110 mm in length
- Tube has 100 markings on its surface, each marking at an interval of 1 mm.
- Internal diameter of tube is 3 mm

b. Pasteur pipette
- It should reach the bottom of Wintrobe tube

c. Centrifuge machine

Specimen: EDTA blood

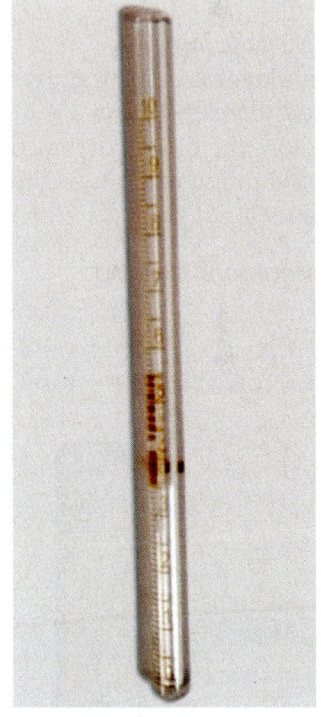

Fig. 18.1: Wintrobe's tube

Methods

- Mix the anticoagulated blood sample thoroughly.
- Draw the blood in Pasteur pipette and introduce the pipette up to the bottom of the Wintrobe tube.
- Fill the tube from the bottom up to 100 mark
- Centrifuge it for 30 minutes

- Take the reading of the length of the column of red cells.
- Hematocrit/PCV is expressed as percentage

Interpretation (Fig. 18.2)
- After centrifugation, following zones are seen in Wintrobe tube from above downwards—plasma, buffy coat layer, and packed red cells.
- Length of the column of red blood cells indicates packed cell volume.
- In anemia, PCV is below the lower level of normal range.
- PCV is raised in dehydration, shock, burns, polycythemia.

Uses of buffy coat layer
- Buffy coat layer is a small grayish layer of WBCs and platelets, about 1 mm thick.
- Smears from the buffy coat layer are used for demonstration of lupus erythematosus (LE) cell, malarial parasite.

2. Microhematocrit Method

Equipment
a. *Microhematocrit centrifuge* should provide a centrifugal force of 12000 g for 5 minutes.

b. *Capillary hematocrit tubes:* Disposable glass tubes 75 mm in length and 1 mm in internal diameter.
c. Tube sealant like plastic sealant or clay
d. Microhematocrit reader or graph paper.

Methods
- Fill the capillary tube by applying its tip to the blood and the tube should be filled with ¾ of its length.
- Seal the other end of capillary tube with sealant
- Centrifuge these tubes
- Remove these tubes from the centrifuge machines and stand them upright.
- Tubes will show three layers from top to bottom: Plasma, buffy coat, column of red cells.

Note: Rules of 3 and 9
PCV = hemoglobin (gm/dl) × 3
PCV = red cell count (million/cu mm) × 9

Reference values of PCV
Adult males: 40–50%
Adult females: 38–45%
Adult females (pregnant): 36–42%
Newborns: 44–60%

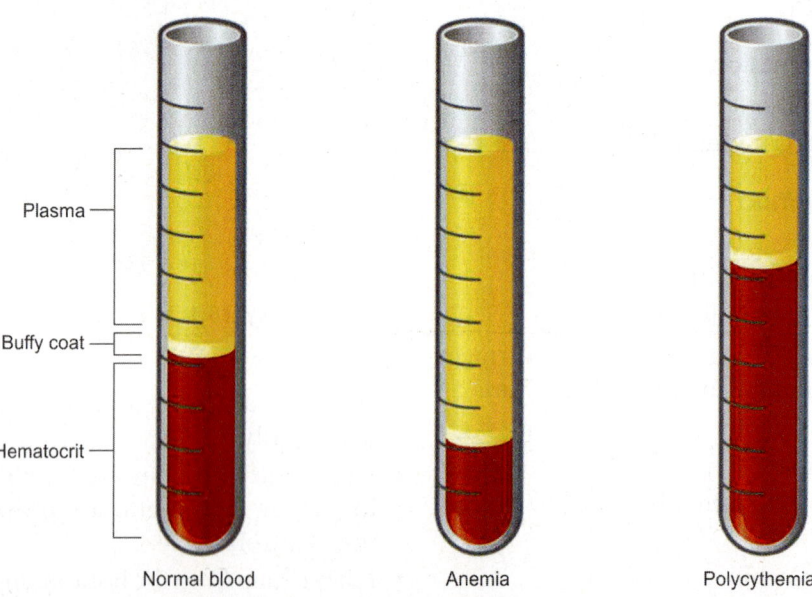

Plasma

Buffy coat

Hematocrit

Normal blood   Anemia   Polycythemia

Fig. 18.2: Packed cell volume assessment

Phlebotomy

- Also called venipuncture
- Procedure of withdrawing blood from a vein.
- And the individual who performs this procedure is called phlebotomist.
- Phlebotomist should be either a doctor, nurse, medical laboratory scientist who are well-trained with the procedure.
- Phlebotomy can be diagnostic or therapeutic
- Diagnostic phlebotomy includes taking the blood samples for hematological, micro-biological or biochemical studies.
- Therapeutic phlebotomy involves taking blood sample as a treatment protocol for hemochromatosis and polycythemia.
- Phlebotomy is done for collection of blood from donors in blood banks.

Venipuncture Sites

Median cubital vein and cephalic veins are most commonly used.

Procedure for Vein Selection

- Palpate and trace the path of veins with the index finger.
- If superficial veins are not seen, it is advisable to force blood into the vein by massaging the arm from wrist to elbow.

Performance of a Venipuncture

- Identify the patient correctly
- Approach the patient in a friendly, calm manner and try to gain the patient's cooperation.
- Properly fill out appropriate requisition forms, indicating the tests ordered.
- Patient's condition should be noted on the lab requisition form, i.e. fasting, dietary restrictions, medications, timing, and medical treatment.
- Check for allergies to antiseptics, adhesives
- Position the patient
- Make the patient sit in a chair, lie down or sit up in a bed.
- Hyperextend the patient's arm
- Apply the tourniquet 3–4 inches above the selected puncture site.
- Do not place too tightly or leave on for more than 2 minutes.
- The patient should make a fist without pumping the hand.
- Select the venipuncture site
- Prepare the patient's arm using an alcohol preparation.
- Cleanse in a circular fashion, beginning at the site and working outward and allow it to air dry.
- Needle should form a 15 to 30° angle with the surface of the arm.
- Insert the needle through the skin and into the lumen of the vein.

- Avoid trauma and excessive probing
- After the sampling is done, remove the tourniquet.
- Remove the needle from the patient's arm
- Press down on the gauze once the needle is out of the arm, applying adequate pressure in order to avoid hematoma formation.

- Dispose of the contaminated material in designated bags.
- Mix and label all appropriate tubes, in which the blood is taken to conduct tests.
- Make sure the samples should reach the laboratory as soon as possible.

Platelets

- Platelets are small, 1–3 microns in diameter, structures with irregular projections on their surface.
- Platelets are produced when the fragments of megakaryocytes are shed in the bone marrow.
- Lifespan of platelet is 7–10 days
- Normal count is 1.5–4.5 lakh/ microliter

Platelet contains two types of cytoplasmic granules

a. *α-Granule components*
  - Have adhesion molecule P-selectin on their membranes.
  - *Proteins involved in coagulation:* Fibrinogen, coagulation factor V, and vWF.
  - *Factors involved in wound healing:* Fibronectin, platelet factor-4, platelet-derived growth factor (PDGF), and transforming growth factor-β.
b. *Dense (or δ) granule components:* Adenosine diphosphate (ADP), adenosine triphosphate, ionized calcium, serotonin, and epinephrine.

Platelets Function

Platelets themselves serve as actual plugs which block the wound. This is achieved by aggregation of platelets at wound site, which blocks the wound and prevents bleeding. This is accomplished through the following steps:
1. *Adhesion:* Platelets sticking around the wound.
2. *Secretion:* Release of their contents of coagulation factors.
3. *Aggregation:* Large numbers of platelets sticking to each other inside the wound thus forming a plug to stop blood flow through the wound.

Thrombocytopenia

Defined as reduction in platelet count.

Causes

a. *Decreased production of platelets*
  - Infections: Measles, HIV
  - Vitamin B_{12}/folate deficiency
  - Leukemia, cancers, myelodysplastic syndromes.
b. *Decreased platelet survival*
  - Immune thrombocytopenic purpura (acute and chronic)
  - Systemic lupus erythematosus
  - B cell lymphomas
  - Drugs: Heparin, quinidine
  - Disseminated intravascular coagulation.

Megakaryopoiesis

- Process concerned with the production of platelets, which take place in bone marrow and result in the release of platelets into peripheral blood.
- Roughly, around 35,000 ± 4300 platelets/ml are made per day.

- Platelets are released into the blood due to the fragmentation of cytoplasm of mega-karyocytes.

Maturational Sequence

Five morphologically identifiable stages of megakaryocytic cells in the bone marrow:

1. *Megakaryoblast:* 15–50 microns in size with blue cytoplasm and nuclei showing fine nuclear chromatin with 1–2 nucleoli.

2. *Pro-megakaryocyte:* 20–80 microns in size with the nucleus showing 2–3 nucleoli.

3. *Granular megakaryocyte:* Cell size varies from 30 to 90 microns, has abundant cytoplasm with reddish blue granules and contains numerous nuclei with coarse nuclear chromatin.

4. *Mature megakaryocyte*
   - Largest cell seen in the bone marrow with abundant cytoplasm.
   - Platelets start breaking up from the cytoplasm into the peripheral blood.

5. *Platelet:* Small fragments of the mega-karyocyte cytoplasm and are of 1–4 microns in size.

Red Cell Indices

Red cell induces include
- Mean corpuscular volume (MCV)
- Mean cell hemoglobin concentration (MCHC)
- Mean cell hemoglobin (MCH)
- Red cell distribution width (RDW)

Uses of Red Cell Indices

- Classification of anemia into normocytic normochromic, microcytic hypochromic or macrocytic anemias.
- Differentiation of iron deficiency anemia (low MCV, MCH and MCHC) from thalassemia trait (low MCV and MCH with normal MCHC).

1. Mean Cell Volume

- Measure of average size of RBCs
- $MCV = \dfrac{PCV\%}{\text{Red cell count in million per mm}^3} \times 100$
- MCV is expressed in femtoliters or fl
- Normal MCV—80–100 fl

Note
- Mentzer's index is derived by dividing MCV with RBC count.

- Index value of less than 13—seen in thalassemia.
- Index value of more than 13—seen in iron deficiency anemia.

2. Mean Cell Hemoglobin (MCH)

- Amount of hemoglobin in a single red blood cell
- $MCH = \dfrac{\text{Hemoglobin in gm\%}}{\text{Red cell in million per mm}^3} \times 100$
- MCH is expressed in picograms or pg
- Normal MCH—27–32 pg

3. Mean Cell Hemoglobin Concentration

- Concentration of hemoglobin in 1 liter of packed red blood cells
- $MCHC = \dfrac{\text{Hemoglobin in gm\%}}{\text{PCV in \%}} \times 100$
- Normal MCHC = 30–35 gm%

4. Red Cell Distribution Width (RDW)

- Measure of degree of variation in red cell size
- Low in beta-thalassemia trait, high in iron deficiency anemia and normal in anemia of chronic disease
- Normal RDW—11.5–14.5

Reticulocyte Count

Reticulocytes (Fig. 22.1)

- Reticulocytes are young RBCs containing remnants of RNA and ribosomes.
- Recognized by supravital stains which detect RNA in these cells.
- RNA appears as blue precipitating granules within RBCs.
- Supravital staining refers to staining of these cells in a living state.

Principle

Few drops of blood are incubated with methylene blue solution which stains granules of RNA in red cells.

Reagent

New methylene blue solution is prepared as follows:

- New methylene blue—1 gm
- Sodium citrate—0.6 gm
- Sodium chloride—0.7 gm
- Distilled water—100 ml

Reagent should be kept stored in a refrigerator at 2–6°C and filtered before use.

Other dyes used include: Brilliant cresyl blue and azure B

Sample: EDTA blood sample.

Methods

1. In a test tube, take 2–3 drops of filtered new methylene blue solution.

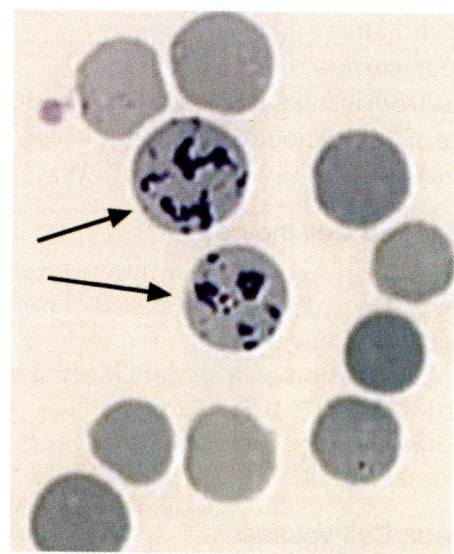

Fig. 22.1: Reticulocytes (arrows)

2. Add equal amount of blood and mix well
3. Keep the mixture at room temperature for 15 minutes.
4. Prepare a smear from the small drop of mixture prepared above.
5. Slide should be viewed under oil immersion lens in a microscope.
6. Reticulocytes show deep blue precipitates in the red blood cells.

Result

Number of reticulocyte is expressed as a percentage of red cells.

Reference Range

Reticulocyte percentage—0.5–2.5%

Increased reticulocyte count (reticulocytosis) is seen in

a. Hemolytic anemia
b. Blood loss
c. Following treatment of nutritional anemia (like iron deficiency, folate deficiency, vitamin B_{12} deficiency)
d. Hemoglobinopathies, e.g. sickle cell anemia

Decreased reticulocyte count (reticulocytopenia) is seen in

a. Aplastic anemia
b. Bone marrow infiltration (leukemia, lymphoma, malignancy)
c. Renal disease
d. Anemia of chronic disease
e. Alcoholism
f. Ineffective erythropoiesis as seen in megaloblastic anemia, thalassemia.
g. Following blood transfusion

Sickling Test

- Red blood cells, which are deprived of oxygen, containing HbS becomes sickle shaped.
- Reducing agent (to remove oxygen from red cells) is 2% sodium metabisulfite.

Procedure

- Drop of capillary or anticoagulated venous blood is mixed on a glass slide with a drop of 2% sodium metabisulfite.
- A coverslip is placed over the mixture and sealed with petroleum jelly/paraffin wax.

- Preparation is examined under the microscope after 30 minutes.
- If sickle cells are not seen, examine the slides again after 2 hours, followed by 24 hours.
- Test is reported negative, if the red cells remain round and positive if red cells become sickle shaped (crescent shaped with pointed ends) or holy-leaf shaped.

Note: It is necessary to perform hemoglobin electrophoresis for confirmation of HbS.

Total Leukocyte Count

- Refers to the number of white blood cells in 1 microliter of blood.
- *Methods of estimation:* Manual or microscopic method, automated method.
- *Purpose:* To detect increase or decrease in total number of white blood cells in the blood.

1. Manual Method

Principles

- Sample of whole blood is mixed with a diluent, which lyses red cells and stains nuclei of the white blood cells.
- White blood cells are counted in a Neubauer counting chamber under the microscope.

Equipment used

a. *Neubauer counting chamber*
   - Composed of ruled areas on the surface of the chamber.
   - Central large square is divided into 25 squares, each of which is divided into 16 small squares.
   - There are surrounding large four corner squares.
   - Four large corner squares are used for counting leukocytes.
   - Central large square is used for counting platelets and red blood cells.
b. Pipette calibrated to deliver 20 microliters (0.02 ml, 20 cu mm)
c. Graduated pipette of 1 ml
d. Pasteur pipette
e. Test tube

Reagents

- Turk's fluid (WBC diluting fluid) consists of glacial acetic acid, which lyses red blood cells and gentian violet, which stains leukocyte nuclei deep violet.
- Composition of Turk's fluid: Glacial acetic acid (2 ml), gentian violet (1 ml), distilled water (100 ml).

Method

Add 0.1 ml of blood into 1.9 ml of diluting fluid, in order to get 1:20 dilution.

2. Charging the Chamber

- Place the coverslip on the Neubauer's chamber.
- Draw some of the diluted blood in a Pasteur pipette.
- Hold the Pasteur pipette at an angle of 45° and place the tip between the coverslip and the chamber.
- The sample should cover the entire ruled area, and should not contain air bubbles.
- Allow 2 minutes for settling of cells.

3. Counting of Cells

- WBCs should be counted on the chamber

- Total cell count = Number of WBCs counted × 50

Normal range: In adults: 4000–11000/mm³

Note: A bulb pipette should not be used for counting WBCs as it is not possible to obtain reliable mixing of blood and diluting fluid inside the bulb of the pipette.

RBC COUNT

- For RBC count, RBC pipette is used, which has a red dot.
- Diluting fluid used for RBC count is Hayem's fluid which is composed of mercuric chloride, sodium sulfate, sodium chloride, distilled water.
- Hayem's fluid results in RBC hemolysis.
- Aspirate the blood up to 0.5 mark of the pipette and the diluting fluid should be aspirated up to 101 mark. Hence, blood specimen is diluted in a ratio of 1:200 with the RBC diluting fluid.
- Hold the pipette horizontally, and roll it with both the hands between the finger and thumb.
- Hold the pipette at an angle of 45° and place the tip between the coverslip and the chamber.
- Allow the cells to settle down for 2 minutes
- Count the total number of cells in the red boxes as depicted in Fig. 24.1.
- After counting the cells, total number of RBCs are calculated as follows.
- N (total number of RBCs/mm³ of blood) = Number of RBCs counted on the chamber × 10000

PLATELET COUNT

Diluting fluid: 1% ammonium oxalate
Principle: 1% ammonium oxalate lyses the red blood cells.

Procedure

- Take 950 microliters of diluting fluid in a clean, dry test tube.
- Add 50 microliters of anticoagulated blood sample and mix.

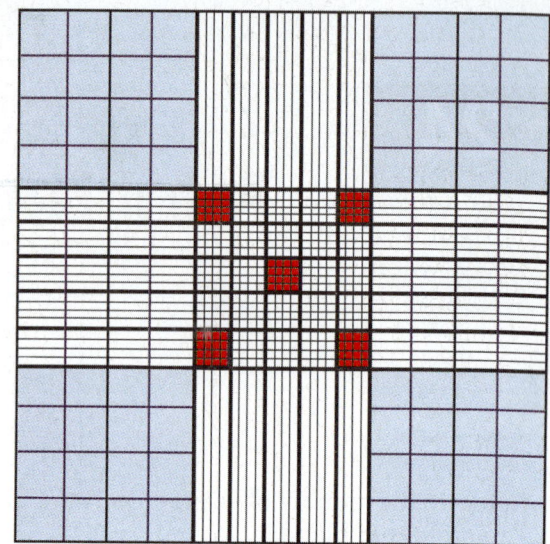

Fig. 24.1: Blue areas: WBCs are counted. Red areas: RBCs/platelets are counted

- Keep for 5 minutes at room temperature
- Mix and fill the chamber with the help of pipette.
- Keep the charged chamber in a moist petri-dish for 5 to 10 minutes and allow the platelets to settle down.
- Count the platelets in the same area as of RBC squares (n).
- Total number of platelets = n × 1000/mm³

EOSINOPHIL COUNT

Diluting fluid: Dunger's fluid
Composition: Eosin yellow—0.5 gm, 95% acetone—0.5 ml, 40% formalin—0.5 ml, distilled water—99 ml.

Principle

Blood is diluted with a diluting fluid, which stains the eosinophilic granules brightly and lyses RBCs and WBCs.

Procedure

- Take 950 microliters of diluting fluid in a clean, dry test tube.
- Add 50 microliters of anticoagulated blood sample and mix.

- Keep for 5 minutes at room temperature
- Mix and fill the chamber with the help of pipette.
- Keep the charged chamber in a moist petridish for 5 to 10 minutes.
- Count the eosinophils under low power (10x) in four corner squares with reduced light (N).
- Absolute eosinophil count = N × 50/mm^3.

Precautions while using Neubauer Counting Chamber

- Preparation of the diluting fluids must be proper.
- Always clean the chamber before and after use.
- After taking blood in pipette clean the outer surface of the tip before diluting it in the diluting fluid.
- Always mix the dilution before filling the chamber.
- Avoid bubbles to come in the chamber
- Never overflow the chamber with dilution
- Change the coverslip, if it is dirty and scratched.
- Calculation must be done properly
- Clean the microscope before and after use.

White Blood Cells (WBCs)

- White blood cells are spherical cells, with a nucleus, and appear white in color as it lacks hemoglobin.
- *Five types of WBCs:* Granulocytes (neutrophils, eosinophils, basophils) and agranulocytes (lymphocytes, monocytes).

Granulocytes (Fig. 25.1)

a. *Neutrophils*
  - 10–12 microns in diameter
  - Nucleus with two to four lobes, connected by thin filaments
  - Reddish purple, cytoplasmic granules
  - *Function:* Phagocytosis and killing of infectious agent.

b. *Basophils*
  - 10–12 microns in diameter
  - Nucleus with two indistinct lobes, cytoplasmic granules stain blue-purple.
  - Releases histamine which promotes inflammation and heparin which prevents clot formation.

c. *Eosinophils*
  - 11–14 microns in diameter
  - Bilobed nucleus, cytoplasmic granules look orange red or bright red.
  - Releases chemical that reduces inflammation and attacks parasites.

d. *Lymphocytes*
  - 6–14 microns in diameter
  - Round nucleus
  - Produces antibodies and other mediators for destroying microorganisms.
  - Plays a role in allergic reactions, graft rejections, tumor control and regulation of immune system.

e. *Monocytes*
  - 12–20 microns in diameter
  - Nucleus appears round, kidney shaped or horseshoe shaped and has abundant cytoplasm.
  - Phagocytic cell in blood and in tissues gets converted to macrophages, which phagocytose bacteria, dead cells and microorganisms.

Normal WBC counts: 4000–11000 cells/mm^3

Differential white blood cell count
- Neutrophils: 40–75%
- Lymphocytes: 20–40%

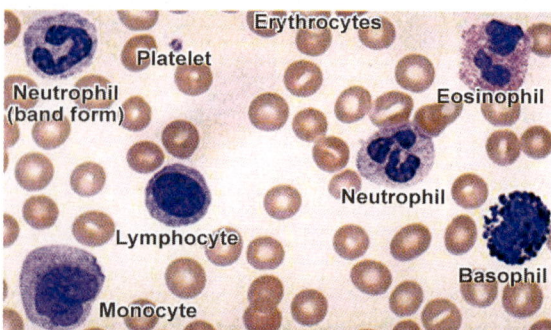

Fig. 25.1: White blood cells in peripheral smear

- Eosinophils: 1–6%
- Monocytes: 2–10%
- Basophils: 0–1%

Leukopenia: Low white cell count (leukopenia)

Neutropenia: Reduction in number of neutrophils in the blood.

Causes

a. *Inadequate production:* Marrow suppression due to tumors, drugs (alkylating agents, antimetabolites) or granulomas.

b. *Increased destruction:* SLE, splenomegaly, bacterial and fungal infections.

Lymphopenia: Reduction in lymphocyte count.

Causes: Human immunodeficiency virus (HIV) infection, corticosteroids, or cytotoxic drugs, autoimmune disorders, malnutrition, acute viral infection.

Leukocytosis: Increase in number of white cells in the blood.

Causes: Chronic infection, myeloproliferative disorders (e.g. chronic myeloid leukemia).

Neutrophilic leukocytosis (increased neutrophil count): Acute bacterial infections.

Eosinophilic leukocytosis (increased eosinophil count): Allergic disorders, parasitic infestations, lymphomas, autoimmune disorders.

Basophilia (increased basophil count): Myeloproliferative disorders.

Monocytosis (increased monocyte count): Tuberculosis, endocarditis, malaria.

Lymphocytosis (increased lymphocyte count): Tuberculosis, viral infections.

Section
II

Histological Techniques

Stains for Amyloid

A. Congo Red Stain for Amyloid

Basis for Congo red method: Congo red is a diazo dye which attaches itself parallel to the amyloid fibrils, the union being affected by H-bond between the –OH groups of amyloid and amino acid groups of the dye.

Preparation of Congo red stain (stock solution)
- 80% ethanol saturated with Congo red and NaCl.
- Allow it to stand for 24 hours before use
- Can be used for months

Working solution
- To 50 ml of the stock solution add 0.5 ml of 1% aqueous NaOH.
- Filter and use within 15 minutes

Procedure
1. Bring the sections to the water
2. Stain with filtered Congo red solution for 25 minutes.
3. Wash in distilled water, followed by running tap water for 5 minutes.
4. Stain with hematoxylin for 1 minute (nuclear stain)
5. Differentiate rapidly in 1% acid alcohol
6. Wash in water
7. Dehydrate, clear and mount

Results
- Amyloid—pink to red
- Nuclei—blue

B. Crystal Violet for Amyloid

Preparation of the solution
- Dissolve 2 gm of crystal violet in 20 ml of 95% alcohol
- Add 80 ml of 1% aqueous ammonium oxalate
- Dissolve with heating
- Cool and filter

Methods
1. Bring the sections to water, remove pigment where necessary
2. Stain in crystal violet solution for 5 minutes
3. Wash and differentiate in weak (0.2%) acetic acid, and check under microscope.
4. After achieving adequate differentiation, rinse the slides in distilled water.
5. Mount with glycerine (Note: DPX should not be used)

Results
- Amyloid—red purple
- Background—blue

Other stains to demonstrate Congo red
a. Hematoxylin and eosin
b. Thioflavin-T

Cryostat

Principles of Frozen Section

- When water in the tissue is frozen, it turns to ice and in this state the tissue is firm.
- Hence, ice acts as an embedding media

Advantage (Fig. 27.1)

It provides a rapid diagnosis.

Consistency of frozen block is hard when temperature is reduced and soft when raised.

Technique

A. *Optimal conditions*
- Block temperature should be correct for the tissue being cut.
- Microtome should be operating correctly
- Anti-roll plate adjustment should be correct.

B. *Anti-roll plate*
- It stops curling up of sections
- Determines the success of sectioning

C. *Points to be considered*
- Correct height to blade angle
- Correct angle to blade
- Top edge should not be damaged
- Optimal cabinet temperature

Applications

- Rapid production of sections for urgent diagnosis. Example: 'On-table' diagnosis of malignancy.
- Diagnostic and research enzyme histo-chemistry.
- Immunofluorescent methods
- Immunocytochemical methods

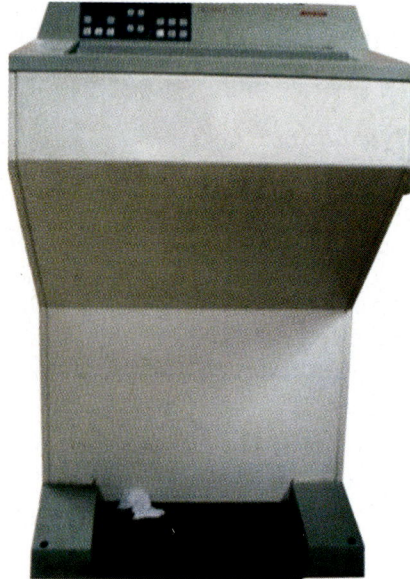

Fig. 27.1: Cryostat

- Diagnostic and research non-enzyme histochemistry
- Example: For lipids and carbohydrates.

Methods of Freezing

a. *Fresh unfixed tissue*
   - Fresh tissue should be frozen as rapidly as possible.
   - Slow freezing will bring tissue distortion
   - Freezing techniques: Liquefied nitrogen, carbon dioxide gas, aerosol sprays.
b. *Fixed tissue*
   - It is preferable for localization of antigens
   - Fixatives used include: (a) Cold acetone for 5 minutes, (b) cold methanol for 5 minutes, (c) 70% ethanol for 15–30 seconds, (d) 4% formaldehyde freshly prepared from paraformaldehyde for 5 minutes, and (e) mixtures from ethanol and formaldehyde.

Section cutting: Very sharp disposable knives should be used.

Cutting speed: Faster stroke is better for harder tissues and slower for softer.

Coated glass slides are used, various coating agents applied on slides are poly-L-lysine, bovine serum albumin.

Staining: Slides are stained with rapid H and E.

Cytochemical Stains

Cytochemistry: Technique for demonstration of enzymes or substances in the cytoplasm of hematopoietic cells.

Types of Cytochemical Stains

1. *Enzymatic:* Myeloperoxidase, non-specific esterase (NSE), phosphatase (leukocyte alkaline phosphatase).
2. *Non-enzymatic:* Sudan black B (SBB), periodic acid-Schiff (PAS), toluidine blue, Perls' stain.

A. Myeloperoxidase (MPO) Stain

- Enzyme presents in primary and secondary granules of neutrophils and its precursors.
- Used to differentiate between myelogenous and monocytic leukemia from acute lymphoblastic leukemia (ALL).

Principle

MPO is present in primary granules and catalyses the oxidative reaction of H_2O_2.

Solutions Required

1. *Solution A*
   - 0.3 gm of benzidine base is dissolved in 99 ml of absolute ethanol.
   - To this, 1 ml of saturated sodium nitro-prusside solution is added.
2. *Solution B*
   - Freshly prepared

- 0.5 ml of H_2O_2 solution is added to 25 ml of distilled water.

Working solution:
- Solution A—5 ml
- Solution B—3 drops

Steps

- Formal vapor fixed smears are taken
- Treat with working solution for 1 minute
- Water wash for 3–4 minutes
- Air dry the smears
- Counterstain with Leishman's stain/ Wright's stain.

Results (Fig. 28.1)

- Myeloblasts in AML show fine to coarse brown cytoplasmic granularity.
- RBCs show diffuse brown positivity and are taken as internal control.

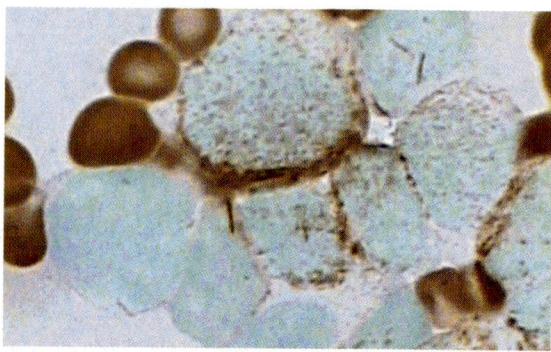

Fig. 28.1: MPO stain demonstrating granular positivity in myeloid precursor cells

B. Sudan Black B (SBB)

Principle

SBB is a lipophilic dye that stains intracellular phospholipids and lipids.

Use

To differentiate between ALL and AML.

Reagents

- Formalin vapors
- 0.3 gm of Sudan black B in 100 ml absolute alcohol.
- *Phenolic buffer:* Phenol in 30 ml of absolute ethanol. Add this to 100 ml distilled water.
- Working stain solution—40 ml of phenolic buffer to 60 ml SBB solution
- Counterstain: Leishman stain.

Procedure

1. Fix air-dried smear in formalin vapors for 5–10 minutes.
2. Air dry for 15 minutes
3. Stain with working solution of SBB for 1 hour.
4. Give 3 washings of ethanol for 30 seconds each.
5. Counterstain with Leishman stain.

Result (Fig. 28.2)

Granules appear black.

C. Periodic Acid–Schiff (PAS)

Principles

- Periodic acid oxidizes 1–2 glycol groups of carbohydrates to produce stable di-aldehydes.
- These dialdehydes give a red reaction product when exposed to Schiff reagent.

Reagents

- Fixative—methanol
- 1% periodic acid
- Schiff's reagent
- Counterstain with hematoxylin

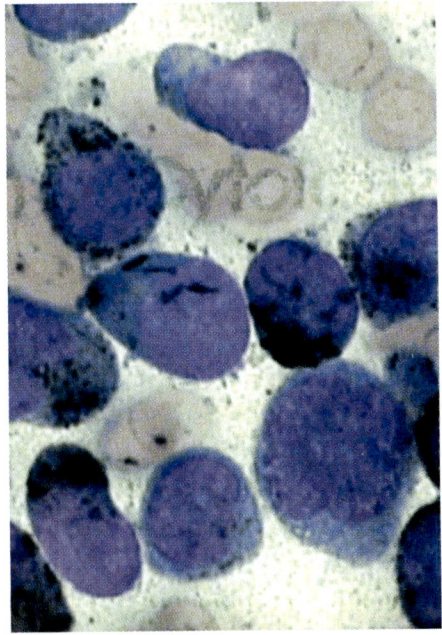

Fig. 28.2: SBB stain demonstrating black granular positivity in myeloid precursors

Procedure

1. Fix slides for 15 minutes in methanol
2. Rinse in running tap water and air dry
3. Treat slides with 1% periodic acid for 10 min
4. Rinse in running tap water for 10 minutes and dry with blot tissue paper (drying is critical step here)
5. Now treat with Schiff's reagent for 10 minutes.

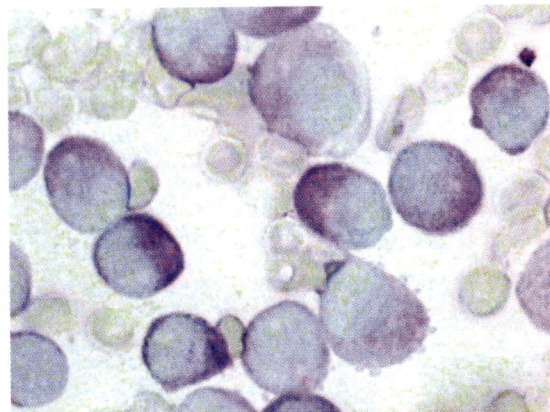

Fig. 28.3: PAS showing diffuse cytoplasmic positivity

6. Rinse in running tap water
7. Counterstain with hematoxylin, then wash and air dry.

Results (Fig. 28.3)

• Reaction product is red
• Cytoplasmic positivity may be diffuse or granular.

• Lymphoblasts are PAS positive
• Monocytes and its precursors are PAS positive.
• Megakaryocytes and blasts are PAS positive.

Note: Also *see* chapter on mucin stains for PAS.

Fixatives

Definition
- Process by which the constituents of cells and tissue are fixed in a physical and chemical state so that they will withstand subsequent treatment with various reagents with minimum loss of architecture.
- Achieved by exposing the tissue to chemical compounds, called fixatives.
- *Volume of fixative:* 15–20 times the volume of the specimen.

Aim of Fixatives
- Preserve cell structure and constituents
- Prevent putrefaction and autolysis
- To stabilize the labile elements, so that they are not lost during subsequent fixation.

What are the Criteria for an Ideal Fixative?
Criteria include
- Rapid penetration and action
- Minimal loss of cell constituents
- Minimal alterations of tissue architecture
- Should be cheap and stable
- Easy to handle
- Should harden the tissues

Effects of fixative
- Causes denaturation, precipitation and cross-linkage of protein.
- With resultant hardening of the tissues

Methods of fixation
- Immersion fixation
- Perfusion fixation
- Vapor fixation
- Coating and spray fixatives
- Microwave fixation

Classification of Fixatives
1. *Based on component*
   a. *Simple fixative:* Formaldehyde, glutaraldehyde.
   b. *Compound fixative:* Carnoy's fixative, Zenker's fluid.
2. *According to action upon cell and tissue*
   a. *Micro-anatomical fixatives:* Neutral formalin, Zenker's fluid.
   b. *Nuclear fixative:* Clarke, Carnoy
   c. *Cytoplasmic fixative:* Champy, formal saline.
   d. *Histochemical fixative:* Acetone, absolute alcohol, neutral buffered formalin.
3. *Based on chemical nature*
   a. *Aldehydes:* Formaldehyde, glutaraldehyde
   b. *Oxidizing agents:* Osmium tetroxide, potassium dichromate.
4. *Protein denaturing agents*
   Alcohol, methyl alcohol, ethyl alcohol
5. *Physical agents*
   Heat and microwaves
6. *Miscellaneous*
   Mercuric chloride, picric acid

Important Fixatives to Remember

1. *Formaldehyde*

- Available as 40% aqueous solution of gas by weight, known as formalin.
- Routinely 10% formalin is used, prepared by mixing 10 ml formaldehyde and 90 ml distilled water.
- *pH:* 6.3–6.5
- *Mechanism of action:* Polymerizes protein molecules by forming methylene bridges.
- *Impurities in formalin:* Methanol, formic acid, paraformaldehyde.

Advantages

1. Rapid penetration
2. Easy availability and cheap
3. Does not over-harden the tissue
4. Fixes lipids for frozen sections

Disadvantages

1. Vapors are irritating
2. Dermatitis
3. Forms formalin pigment in tissues with high vascularity.

2. *Glutaraldehyde*

- Fixative of choice for electron microscopy
- Used as 2.5–4% solution
- Should be stored in refrigerator at 4°C
- More efficient cross-linking
- Less shrinkage but more expensive
- Does not fix lipids

3. *Alcohol Fixative*

- Includes absolute alcohol, ethanol, methanol, Carnoy's fixative, Clarke's fluid.
- *Mechanism:* Denatures and precipitates proteins.
- *80–100% methyl alcohol:* Used as an excellent fixative for dry and wet smears.
- Ethyl alcohol: Fixative for enzymes

Carnoy's fixative contains

- Ethanol—60 ml
- Chloroform—30 ml
- Glacial acetic acid—10 ml

Fixation time 1–3 hours

- Preserves glycogen and rapid fixation for small biopsies
- Ideal for lymph node fixation

Clarke's fluid contains

- Methanol and glacial acetic acid
- Good nuclear fixative

Osmium tetroxide: Used in neurohistology and neuropathology.

Potassium dichromate: Demonstration of mitochondria, Golgi apparatus, mitotic figures, chromaffin cells.

4. *Picric Acid Fixatives*

Bouin's fluid contains:

- Picric acid—75 ml
- Formalin—25 ml
- Glacial acetic acid—5 ml

Fixation time—6 hours

Good fixative for glycogen demonstration.

5. *Mercury Containing Fixative*

Includes Zenker's fixative, Helly's fixative, Heidenhain's fixative and Suza's fixative.

Zenker's fluid

- Distilled water—950 ml
- Potassium dichromate—25 g
- Mercuric chloride—50 g
- Glacial acetic acid—50 g

Fixation time: 4–24 hours

- Fixed tissue should be washed overnight in running tap water before processing.
- Excellent for connective tissue fibers.

Factors Affecting Fixation

1. *pH:* Satisfactory fixation occurs at pH 6–8
2. *Temperature*
   - Fixation is carried out at room temperature
   - High temperature fixation is used for urgent biopsies.

- Low temperature fixation is required for electron microscopy and histochemistry.
3. *Penetration:* Rate of penetration is 1 mm/hour
4. *Agitation:* It increases the speed of penetration
5. *Osmolarity*
   - Hypertonic solutions: Cell shrinkage
   - Hypotonic and isotonic fixatives: Cell swelling
6. *Size:* Ideal size of the tissue should be 3–4 mm.

7. *Time*
   - Minimum fixation time for tissue up to 5 mm in thickness is 12 hours.
   - Prolonged fixation can cause shrinkage and hardening of the tissue and severe inhibition of enzyme activity.

Special Fixative used in Cytology

a. *Saccomanno's fixative*
   - 50% alcohol and 2% carbowax
   - For prefixation of sputum

Hematoxylin and Eosin Stain

Hematoxylin stains the cell nuclei blue, black, whereas eosin stains cell cytoplasm pink, orange or red.

Hematoxylin

- Extracted from the tree *Haematoxylon campechianum.*
- Its major oxidation product, i.e. hematein, is responsible for its color.
- Hematein can be produced from hematoxylin either by natural oxidation (exposure to light or air) or chemical oxidation.
- Chemical oxidation is done by using sodium iodate (e.g. in Mayer's hematoxylin) and mercuric oxide (e.g. in Harris's hematoxylin).
- Hematein is anionic and does not stain anionic nuclei without a mordant.
- *Mordant:* Results in cationic charge on the hematein molecule, which now can bind to the anionic site, i.e. nuclear chromatin, e.g. aluminum, iron, tungsten.
- Hematoxylin can be classified according to the mordant used: Alum hematoxylin, iron hematoxylin, tungsten hematoxylin, molybdenum hematoxylin, lead hematoxylin.

Alum Hematoxylin

- Mordant used is aluminum
- Stains the nuclei a red color

Definition

- Oxidizing agent—used to begin the ripening process that helps to transform hematoxylin to hematin, e.g. sodium iodate, HgO_2.
- Mordant—substance responsible for induction of color in a dye, e.g. aluminum sulphate/ alum.

Bluing

- Method by which the red color of nuclei is converted to blue black, occurs when a section is washed in a weak alkali solution.
- Tap water is alkaline and can bring this color change.
- *Other solutions used are:* Lithium carbonate, ammonia in distilled water, Scott's tap water.

Types of Staining

- *Progressive staining:* Section is stained for a predetermined time for adequate staining of nuclei, e.g. Mayer's hematoxylin, Gill's hematoxylin.
- *Regressive staining:* Section is over-stained and then differentiated in acid alcohol followed by bluing, e.g. Harris hematoxylin, Delafield's hematoxylin, Ehrlich's hematoxylin.

Preparation of Solution

Hematoxylin
- Hematoxylin: 2.5 gm
- Absolute alcohol: 25 ml
- Potassium alum: 50 gm
- Distilled water: 500 ml
- Mercuric oxide: 1.25 gm

Eosin
Working solution: 1 gm eosin + 100 ml distilled water

Staining Procedure

1. De-wax the sections, rehydrate through the descending grades of alcohol to water.
2. Stain with hematoxylin for 5–15 minutes
3. Wash with running tap water
4. Differentiate in 1% acid alcohol for 5–10 seconds.
5. Wash in running tap water for 20 minutes
6. Stain with eosin for 1 minute
7. Dehydrate through ascending grades of alcohol.
8. Clear in xylene and mount with DpX

Results (Fig. 30.1)

- Nuclei: Blue/black

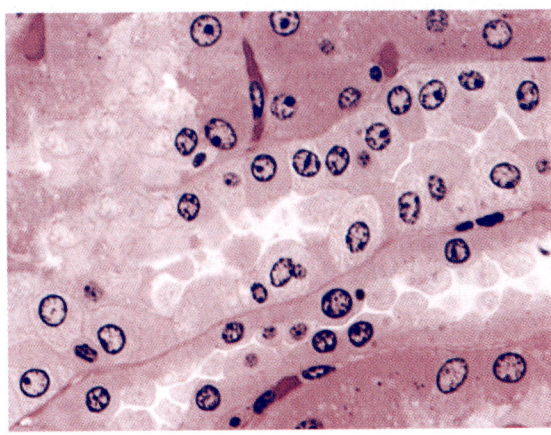

Fig. 30.1: H & E stain slide

- Cytoplasm: Pink
- Muscle fibers: Deep pink/red
- Red blood cells: Orange/red
- Fibrin: Deep pink

Quality Control in H & E Stain

- Care should be taken in steps of fixation, processing schedules, section thickness, excessive hot-plate temperatures.
- New batch staining should be compared to old batch staining for efficacy.

31

Masson-Fontana Silver Stain

Solutions Required

1. *Silver nitrate solution (Fontana)*
   Stock solution: Dissolve 10 gm of silver nitrate in 100 ml of distilled water
   Working solution:
   a. To 1 ml of silver nitrate add ammonium hydroxide drop wise, till it becomes clear
   b. Make the above solution 10 ml by adding distilled water
   c. Keep overnight
2. *Gold chloride solution*
   - 1% aqueous gold chloride—10 ml
   - Distilled water—40 ml
3. *5% sodium thiosulfate solution:* 5 gm of sodium thiosulphate in 100 ml of water.
4. Nuclear fast red solution/eosin solution.

Procedure

1. Deparaffinize and bring the sections to water.
2. Treat the sections with silver nitrate solutionand keep them under light source like sunlight for 1 hour (sections should turn light brown).
3. Rinse in distilled water
4. Treat the sections with gold chloride solution for 10 minutes.
5. Rinse in water for 3 minutes
6. Treat the sections with sodium thiosulfate solution for 5 minutes.
7. Water wash
8. Counterstain with nuclear fast red or aqueous eosin Y for 5 minutes.
9. Dehydrate, clear and mount

Results

- Melanin, argentaffin, chromaffin, lipofuscins black
- Nuclei—pink

Microbial Staining

A. Gram Stain

Technique
1. Deparaffinize and bring the sections to water
2. Add 1–2 ml of crystal violet stain for 1 minute
3. Water wash
4. Gram's iodine solution for 2 minutes
5. Water wash
6. Acetone for 10 seconds
7. Dilute safranine for 1 minute
8. Dry and mount

Results

Gram-positive organism: Blue
Gram-negative organism: Pink

B. Ziehl-Neelsen Stain (for TB Bacilli)

Carbol fuscin stock solution
- Basic fuscin: 1 gm
- Absolute alcohol: 10 ml
- 50% aqueous phenol: 90 ml

Steps

1. Deparaffinize and bring the sections to water.
2. Treat the sections with preheated carbol fuscin solution for 20 minutes.
3. Wash with water
4. Decolorize it with 20% H_2SO_4
5. Counterstain with Löffler's methylene blue for 30 seconds.
6. Dehydrate with alcohol
7. Clear with Xylene
8. Mount with DPX.

Results

- AFB—red
- Nuclei—blue
- Other tissue constituents—pale blue
- Nocardia filaments—red
- Lipofuscin—red

C. Fite-stain for Lepra Bacilli

Materials
1. Xylene—turpentine oil:
   - Turpentine oil—1 part
   - Xylene—2 parts
2. Carbol fuscin solution:
   - Basic fuscin—4 gm
   - Phenol crystal melted—8 ml
   - 95% alcohol—20 ml
   - Distilled water—100 ml
   Note: Filter before use
3. 3% sulfuric acid solution
   - Concentrated sulfuric acid—3 ml
   - Distilled water—100 ml
4. Methylene blue solution (stock)
   - Methylene blue—1.4 gm
   - 95% alcohol—100 ml
5. Methylene blue solution (working)
   - Methylene blue (stock)—10 ml
   - Tap water—90 ml

Steps

1. Deparaffinize with Xylene-oil mixture.
2. Treat the sections with xylene-oil mixture for 20 minutes.
3. Blot dry with tissue paper
4. Treat with carbol fuscin for 15–20 minutes
5. Wash with water
6. Decolorize with 3% H_2SO_4
7. Rinse in water
8. Counterstain with methylene blue (30 seconds)
9. Rinse in water
10. Alcohol (few seconds)
11. Xylene
12. Mount in DpX

Results

- AFB—red
- Nuclei—blue
- Other tissue constituents—pale blue
- Nocardia filaments—red
- Lipofuscin—red

Points to Remember

- Coating of the microorganisms by turpentine oil and xylene provides protection to the microbial wall.
- Coating is not dissolved when the tissues are treated with alcohol.

Microtomy

Uses

- Required for tissue sectioning
- In order for tissue visualization under the microscope
- Instrument used is called microtome

Types of Microtome

- Rotary
- Rocking
- Base sledge

- Rotary rocking
- Sliding
- Freezing
- Vibrating
- Ultra microtome

A. Rotary Microtome (Fig. 33.1)

- It has a rotary wheel that brings about the cutting movement.
- Knife position is fixed to the microtome.

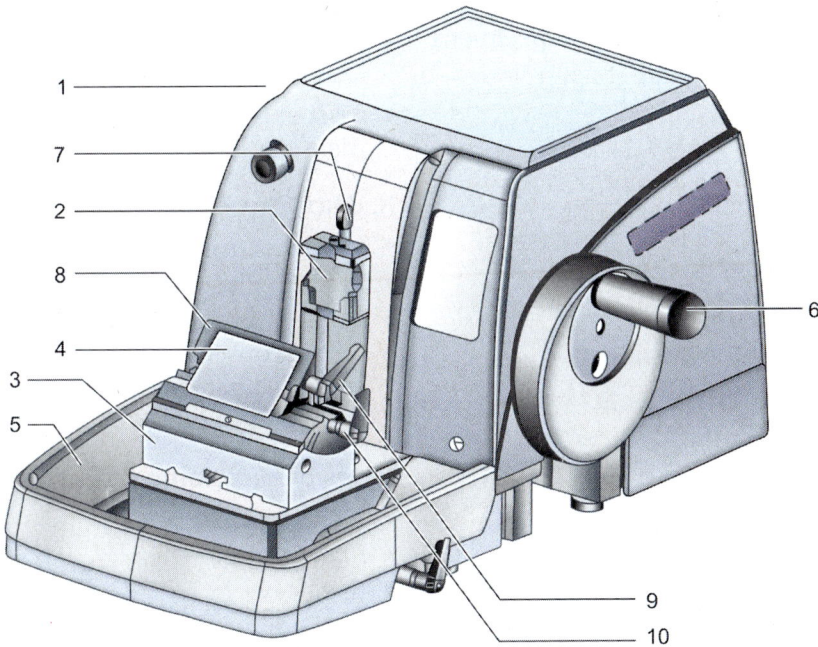

Fig. 33.1: 1. Rotary microtome, 2. block holder, 3. stage mount, 4, 8. knife and its holder, 5. waste tray, 6. rotary arm, 7. block adjustment lever, 9. knife locking lever, 10. knife angle locking lever

Advantages
- Heavier and more stable
- Cuts good accurate sections
- Hard tissues are cut without vibration
- Serial sections can be taken
- Only microtome used for teaching purposes.

Disadvantage
Finger being cut while sectioning.

B. Rocking Microtome
Knife is fixed

Advantages
- Cuts very small blocks, any type of tissue
- Cheap, reliable, easy to maintain

Disadvantages
- Block size to be cut is limited
- Light weight so serrations are seen due to vibrations.

C. Base Sledge Microtome (Fig. 33.2)
Advantages
- Cuts very hard and large blocks
- Neurology and ophthalmology specimens
- Knife-fixed, large wedge shaped
- Knife holder-adjustable

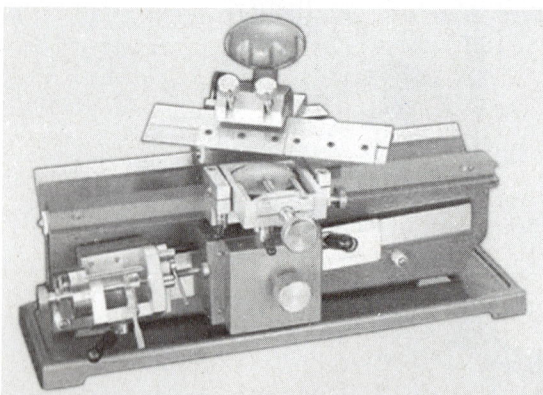

Fig. 33.2: Base sledge microtome

Disadvantage
Consistent 3 mm sections are difficult to produce.

D. Rotary Rocking Microtome
- More robust than the rocking microtome
- Produces a flat face to the tissue block
- *Use:* Cryostat

E. Sliding Microtome
Knife or blade is stationary, the specimen slides under it during sectioning.

F. Freezing Microtome
- Demonstrates fat histologically
- Used for cutting thin to semi-thin sections of fresh frozen tissue.

G. Vibrating Knife Microtome
- Designed to cut fresh unfixed tissue
- High speed vibration is produced in a safety razor blade that provides the cutting power.
- Sections are thicker

Advantages
- Greatest application in enzyme histochemistry and ultrastructure histochemistry.
- Tissues are cut at a very slow speed to avoid disintegration.

H. Ultra Microtome
- Used exclusively for electron microscopy
- Prepare ultrathin sections
- Block is brought to the knife edge under microscopy control and as each section is cut, it is floated onto a water bath adjacent to the knife edge.

Types of Microtome Knives
- Planoconcave
- Plane wedge
- Biconcave
- Tool edge

Classification of Pigments

A. Exogenous Pigments

- Coal dust
- Tattooing

B. Endogenous Pigments

- Lipofuscin
- Melanin
- Ochronosis
- Hemosiderin
- Bile pigment

MINERAL AND PIGMENT STAINING

A. Perls' Stain for Iron

Principle

Potassium ferrocyanide converts hemosiderin (ferrous form), present in the macrophages to ferric ferrocyanide which imparts a blue color to these macrophages.

Fixation

Fix in methanol for 10–20 minutes and dry the slides.

Solution Required

1. 2% potassium ferrocyanide
2. 2% HCl
   Take equal quantities of these two solutions.

Methods

1. Deparaffinize and bring the sections to water
2. Rinse in distilled water
3. Place the slides in equal quantities of potassium ferrocyanide and HCl at room temperature for 20–25 minutes.
4. Wash in running tap water for 5 minutes
5. Counterstain with eosin for 10–15 seconds
6. Dehydrate, clear and mount with DPX

Results

- Iron pigments (hemosiderin)—bright blue
- Nucleus—red
- Cytoplasm—light pink

B. Von Kossa Stain for Calcium

Principle

This method depends on the reaction of the tissue sections with silver nitrate. Tissue containing calcium phosphate (present in the mineral phase of the bone) on reaction with silver nitrate, results in formation of a compound, i.e. silver phosphate.

Procedure

1. Bring the sections to the water
2. Flood the slides with 5% silver nitrate solution and keep it for 1 hour.
3. Wash in several changes of distilled water
4. Treat the sections with gold chloride for 2–3 minutes.
5. Rinse with water
6. Treat with sodium thiosulfate solution for 5 minutes

7. Rinse with water
8. Counter stain with neutral red
9. Dehydrate, clear and mount

Results

- Calcium deposits/bone—black
- Osteoid—red

C. Stain for Bile

Solutions

A. *Fouchet's reagent*
- 25% aqueous trichloroacetic acid
- 10% aqueous ferric chloride
Stain has to be prepared freshly before use.
B. *van Gieson stain:* Dissolve 100 mg of acid fuscin in 100 ml of saturated aqueous picric acid.

Methods

1. Bring the sections to the water
2. Treat with freshly prepared Fouchet's solution for 10–15 minutes.
3. Wash well in running tap water
4. Rinse in distilled water
5. Counterstain with van Gieson solution for 2 minutes.
6. Dehydrate, clear and mount with DPX.

Results

- Bile pigment: Emerald blue-green
- Muscle: Yellow
- Collagen: Red

How Artifactual Formalin and Malaria Pigments are Removed from the Tissue Sections?

A. *Removal of formalin pigment*
- Alcoholic ammonia solution:
  – 50 ml ethanol + 15 ml ammonia

Procedure
1. Bring the sections to water
2. Immerse sections in alcoholic ammonia solution for 1 hour at room temperature.
3. Wash in running tap water

B. *Removal of malarial pigment*
Saturated alcoholic picric acid solution: Saturated picric acid in ethanol solution.

Procedure
1. Bring the sections to the water
2. Immerse the sections in saturated alcoholic picric acid solution for 12–24 hours at room temperature.
3. Wash with running tap water till it removes the yellow color of picric acid.

Mucin Stains

A. PAS Stain

Principles

- Periodic acid oxidizes the compounds having free hydroxyl groups.
- As a result the –OH between the carbon atoms is broken, resulting in production of dialdehyde structure.
- This dialdehyde structure reacts strongly with Schiff's reagent to give a magenta-colored complex.

Routinely used Fixatives for PAS Stain

Formalin for histopathology and methanol fixed slides for peripheral smear and bone marrow slides.

Fixatives of Choice

Zenker's solution, Bouin's solution, Carnoy's solution.

Preparation of Schiff's Reagent

- Boil 200 ml of distilled water in a flask and add 1 gm of basic fuscin and dissolve it.
- Heat the solution to 50°C and add 2 gm of potassium metabisulfite with mixing.
- Cool the solution further to room temperature.
- Add 2 ml of concentrated HCl and mix thoroughly.
- Add 2 gm of activated charcoal, keep overnight in dark, and then filter it.

- Filtrate should be clear or pale in color
- Store at 4°C in dark bottle

Staining Procedure

1. Deparaffinise and bring the sections to the water.
2. Treat the sections with 1% periodic acid solution for 10 minutes. 1% periodic acid is prepared by adding 1 gm of periodic acid in 100 ml of distilled water.
3. Water wash for 10 minutes
4. Treat the sections with Schiff reagent for 10 minutes.
5. Water wash for 5 minutes
6. Counterstain with Harris hematoxylin for 1 minute.
7. Dehydrate, clear and mount.

Results

- Glycogen, neutral/sialomucins and glyco-proteins—magenta color
- Nuclei—blue color

Uses of PAS Stain

- To identify fungi
- For identifying glycogen in glycogen storage disorders, e.g. Gaucher's disease.
- To demonstrate signet ring cells in adeno-carcinomas.

- Diagnosis of leukemia (lymphoblasts in ALL, erythroblasts and megakaryoblasts in AML, both show PAS positivity).
- PAS positive pigments like lipofuscin

Note: Also see chapter on cytochemical stains for PAS stain.

2. Mucicarmine Stain

Ia. *Southgate's mucicarmine stock solution*
- Carmine (alum lake)—1 gm
- Aluminum hydroxide—1 gm
- 50% ethanol—100 ml
- Mix by shaking

b. Then add 0.5 gm of anhydrous aluminum chloride to the above solution.

c. Place the flask in a boiling water bath for 3 minutes and agitate while boiling.

d. Cool the flask under running tap water

e. Filter and store at 4°C

Note: This stock solution is stable for several months.

II. *Mucicarmine working solution*

a. 10 ml of Southgate's mucicarmine stock solution

b. 90 ml of distilled water

III. *Weigert's iron hematoxylin working solution*

a. Alcoholic hematoxylin—50 ml

b. Acidified ferric chloride solution—50 ml

Note: This solution should be used just before use in equal quantities of solutions a and b.

IV. *Metanil yellow working solution*

a. Metanil yellow—0.25 gm

b. Distilled water—100 ml

c. Glacial acetic acid—0.25 ml

Mix and store in a brown bottle or a bottle completely wrapped with aluminum foil.

Staining Procedure

1. Deparaffinize and hydrate in distilled water.
2. Stain in working Weigert's hematoxylin for 5 minutes.
3. Wash in running tap water for 10 minutes

4. Place in diluted mucicarmine working solution for 30–60 minutes.
5. Rinse quickly in distilled water
6. Stain with metanil yellow for 2 minutes
7. Rinse quickly in distilled water
8. Rinse quickly in 95% alcohol
9. Dehydrate in 2 changes of absolute alcohol, clear with 2–3 changes of xylene and mount.

Results

- Mucin: Deep red (magenta, pink)
- Nuclei: Black
- Other tissue elements: Light yellow

Principle

Aluminum is believed to form a chelation complex with carmine and this positively charged carmine aluminum complex binds to negatively charged acidic mucins to give a deep red (magenta, pink) color.

3. Alcian Blue (pH 2.5%)

- Alcian blue—1 gm
- 3% acetic acid—100 ml.

Procedure

1. Dewax the sections, bring it to water
2. Rinse in 3% acetic acid (2 changes)
3. Alcian blue stain: 15 minutes
4. Blot dry
5. Counterstain with 0.5% neutral red for 3 minutes or eosin for 1 minute
6. Wash with water
7. Dehydrate with alcohol for 3 minutes
8. Xylene
9. Mount

Results

- Acid mucin—blue
- Nucleus—red

4. Alcian Blue PAS Sequence (pH 2.5)

1. Bring the sections to water
2. Stain with freshly filtered 1% alcian blue in 3% acetic acid (pH 2.5) for 15 minutes.
3. Wash in water for 5 minutes

4. Oxidize in 1% aqueous periodic acid solution for 10 minutes.
5. Wash in water for 10 minutes
6. Treat with Schiff's reagent for 10 minutes
7. Water wash for 10 minutes
8. Counterstain with hematoxylin for 5 minutes
9. Dehydrate, clear and mount.

Results

Acid mucopolysaccharides, connective tissue mucin: Stained blue (AB positive, PAS negative).

Epithelial mucin, cartilage: Blue-purple (AB and PAS both positive).

Museum Techniques

All teaching laboratories of medical colleges have museums for teaching purposes.

What are the Basic Museum Techniques?

Any specimens for museum are handled by following steps:
1. Reception
2. Preparation
3. Fixation
4. Restoration
5. Preservation
6. Presentation

1. Reception of the Specimen

- All the specimens received in the lab should be recorded in the reception book.
- After receiving, each specimen is given a number followed by the year, e.g. specimen number 18 received for the year 2018 should be labeled as 18/2018.
- The number should be labeled properly on the paper and paper should be firmly attached or stitched to the specimen.
- Reception book should contain all the necessary information about the specimen like clinical, gross and microscopic findings.

2. Preparation of the Specimen

If the specimen has to be mounted, one-half of the specimen should be left undisturbed following its histopathological examination, e.g. kidney can be bisected and one-half kept aside for museum.

3. Fixation of the Specimen

- *Objective:* To preserve the morphology of the cells and tissue constituents.
- Fixatives used in museums are based on formalin fixation techniques and are derived from Kaiserling technique and its modifications.
- Kaiserling recommended that the initial fixation should be a neutral formalin (KI) solution, which is then transferred to a final preserving glycerin solution (KIII)

Kaiserling's Technique
Fixation of the Specimen

- Specimen should be kept in a container which can accommodate the specimen along with 3–4 times the volume of the fixative.
- Specimen is stored in Kaiserling I solution for 1 month.
- Specimen should not rest on bottom of the container in order to prevent the formation of an artificial flat surface, which is formed due to hardening of the tissue (because of fixation).

Kaiserling I Solution

- Formalin—1 litre
- Potassium acetate—45 gm
- Potassium nitrate—25 gm
- Distilled water—make up to 10 litres

Kaiserling II Solution

- For restoration of the color of the specimens, which has been lost due to fixation.
- Specimens removed from Kaiserling I solution are now kept in 95% alcohol for 10 minutes to 1 hour depending on the size of specimen.
- Color restoration takes about 1–1.5 hours, which is restored with the help of rejuvenator solution.
- Rejuvenator solution comprises 100 ml of pyridine, 100 gm of sodium hydrosulphite and 4 litres of distilled water.

Kaiserling III Solution

- The solution, in which the specimen will remain for display.
- For preservation of the specimen
- Based on glycerine solution.

Constituents of the Solution

- Potassium acetate—1416 gm
- Glycerine—4 litres
- Distilled water—make up to 10 liters
- Thymol crystals are added to prevent moulds.

Leave the solution to stand for 2–3 days before using to ensure proper mixing of chemicals.

All museum specimens are mounted in rectangular glass jars (Fig. 36.1) and are covered by rectangular glass plates.

4. Mounting of the Specimens (Fig. 36.2)

- In a jar, specimen is attached to the specimen plate or rectangular bent glass rods.
- It is achieved by tying the specimen with nylon threads.
- Double knots should be made by threads on the specimen surface.

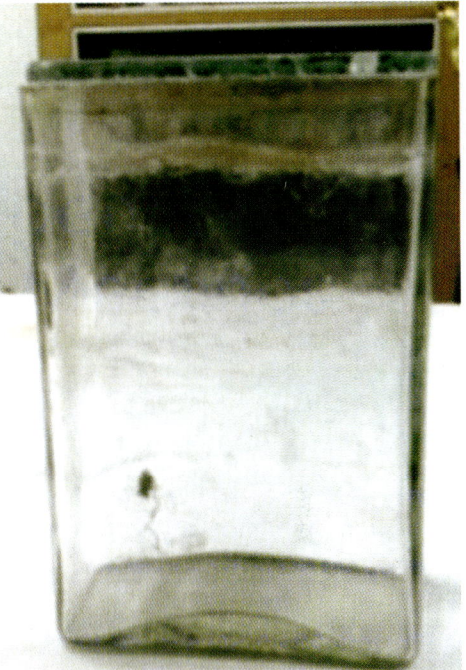

Fig. 36.1: Jar for mounting

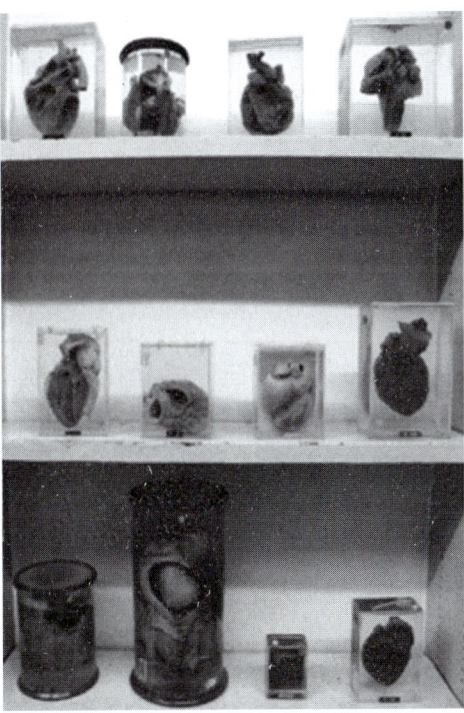

Fig. 36.2: Mounted museum specimens

37

Oil Red O Stain

Use

For neutral lipids.

Solution

- 70% alcohol and 1 pinch of Oil red powder
- Mix thoroughly for 2 minutes

Procedure

1. Treat the smears with this solution for 5–15 minutes.
2. Wash in water
3. Hematoxylin for 1–2 minutes
4. Treat with glycerin and mount

Note: Staining has to be performed on fresh unfixed tissues as alcohol fixation removes lipids.

Result

Oil red O provides red color to the lipids in the tissue.

38

Pap (Papanicolaou) Stain

Reagents

a. *Harris hematoxylin*

- Hematoxylin—5 gm
- Aluminum sulfate—100 gm (mordant)
- Ethyl alcohol—50 ml
- Distilled water—1000 ml
- Mercuric oxide—2.5 gm (oxidizing agent)

b. *Orange G6*

- 10% aqueous orange G—50 ml
- Alcohol—950 ml
- Phosphotungstic acid—0.15 gm

c. *EA-65*

- Alcoholic stock solution of light green—180 ml
- Alcoholic stock solution of Bismarck brown—40 ml
- Alcoholic stock solution of eosin yellow—180 ml
- Phosphotungstic acid—2.4 gm

Filter all stains before use.

Methods

1. Fix the smears in 95% alcohol for 30 minutes
2. Bring the smears to 80% alcohol for 1 minute
3. Bring the smears to 70% alcohol for 1 minute
4. Bring the smears to 50% alcohol for 1 minute
5. Rinse in water for 1 minute
6. Stain in Harris hematoxylin for 5 minutes
7. Rinse in water for 2 minutes
8. Differentiate in 0.5% aqueous HCl for 10 seconds
9. Blue in Scott's tap water for 2 minutes
10. Dehydrate in 70% alcohol for 2 minutes
11. Dehydrate in 95% alcohol for 2 minutes
12. Stain in OG-6 for 2 minutes
13. Bring the smears to 95% alcohol for 2 minutes
14. Stain with EA-65 for 3 minutes
15. Bring the smears to 95% alcohol for 1 minute
16. Acetone (dehydration)
17. Xylene (clearing agent)
18. Air dry the smears
19. Clear and mount with DPX.

Results (Fig. 38.1)

- Nuclei—blue/black
- Cytoplasm (non-keratinizing)—blue/green, keratinizing cells—pink/orange
- RBCs—orange/pink

1. Unsatisfactory Nuclear Staining

A. Nuclear Staining too Pale

1. Contamination of hematoxylin
2. Increased differentiation by HCl
3. Air drying of smears
4. Loss of nuclear material
5. Expiry date of the nuclear stain overlooked
6. Inadequate bluing
7. Inadequate time in hematoxylin

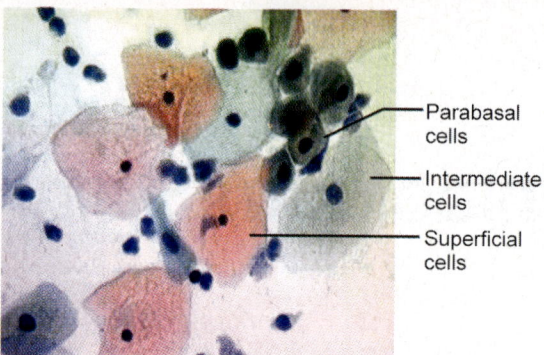

Parabasal cells

Intermediate cells

Superficial cells

Fig. 38.1: Normal Pap smear (satisfactory staining)

B. Nuclear Staining too Dark

1. Prolonged fixation
2. Few dips in HCl

3. Increased concentration of dye
4. High alcohol concentration

2. Unsatisfactory Cytoplasmic Staining

a. Too long dipping in alcohol after cytoplasmic stains
b. Air dry artifact

Contamination Control

1. Stains filtered daily
2. Alcohol and xylene filtered and replaced daily.
3. Gynecology and non-gynecology smears should be stained separately.
4. Urine and other fluids should be stained in separate containers.

Romanowsky Stain

Romanowsky stain contains a combination of acidic dyes and basic dyes.

Acidic dye includes eosin Y

Basic dye includes methylene blue

Acidic dyes are negatively charged and bind to the cationic site and impart orange-red color to hemoglobin and eosinophil granules.

Basic dyes are positively charged and bind to the anionic sites and impart blue color to nuclear acids, basophilic granules.

Examples of Romanowsky stains: Leishman's stain, May-Grunwald-Giemsa sain, Jenner stain, Wright's stain, Field's stain.

Methyl alcohol in these stains acts as a solvent as well as fixative.

These stains have a tendency toward precipitation and should be filtered before use.

A. Leishman's Stain (Fig. 39.1)

Components

Leishman's stain contains methylene blue and eosin dissolved in absolute methyl alcohol.

Preparation

- Commercially available Leishman powder is mixed with methyl alcohol.
- Weigh around 0.2 gm of powder and add to conical flask, followed by addition of 100 ml of methanol and warm the mixture

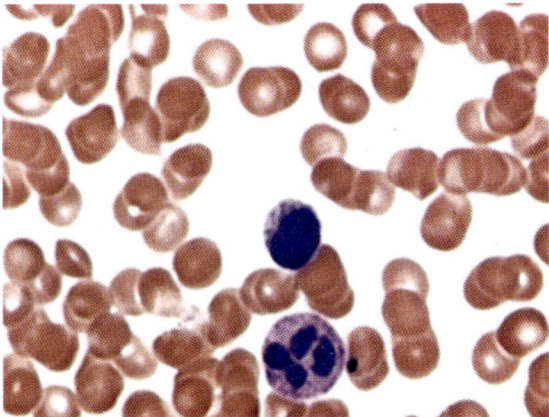

Fig. 39.1: Peripheral smear using Leishman stain

at 50° for 15 minutes. Allow the flask to cool and filter.
- Freshly prepared solution is kept tightly in a brown bottle and stored in a cool, dark place at a room temperature.
- Exposure to the sunlight, will destroy the stain, and stain should be kept for 3–5 days before using as it improves the quality of the stain.

B. May-Grunwald-Giemsa Stain

Fixative: Methanol

Preparation

a. *May-Grunwald stain* (Fig. 39.2)
   - Take May-Grunwald stain powder (0.3 gm) in 100 ml of methanol

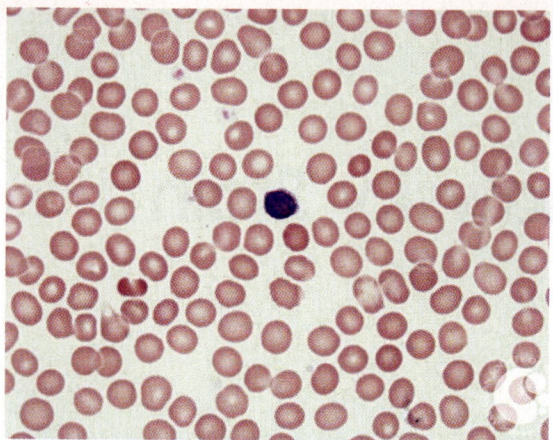

Fig. 39.2: Peripheral smear using May-Grunwald-Giemsa stain

- Dissolve it by rotating and heat up to 50°
- Keep it overnight, filter it and use
- It does not require ripening

b. *Giemsa stain*
- Take 1 gm of powder dye in 100 ml of methanol
- Filter the solution and it is ready for use

Methods
- For May-Grunwald solution, a 1:1 dilution with distilled water is made, which is now poured on the desired slide for 10 minutes.
- For Giemsa, 1:4 dilution with distilled water is prepared.
- Pour off the May-Grunwald solution from the slide and now Giemsa stain is poured on for 20 minutes.

- Wash with distilled water and pour the distilled water on the slide for 2 minutes.
- Make it air dry, mount with DPX.

Results
- Nuclear chromatin appears purple
- RBCs: Red or pink
- Reticulocytes: Gray-blue
- Neutrophils: Pink cytoplasm, purple granules
- Eosinophils: Pale pink cytoplasm, orange red granules
- Basophils: Blue cytoplasm, dark blue-violet granules
- Monocyte: Gray-blue cytoplasm, fine red granules
- Small lymphocyte: Dark blue cytoplasm
- Platelets: Purple

C. Field's Stain
Materials
- Methanol (absolute)
- Field's stain A and B
- Tube with water
- Staining dishes
- Filter paper

Procedure
a. Fix thin film with methanol for 1 min.
b. Dry microscopic slide on filter paper
c. Immerse slide in Field's stain B (eosin) for 5 seconds
d. Immediately wash with water
e. Immerse slide in Field's stain A (methylene blue) for 10 sec
f. Dry thin films.

Stains used for Collagen Demonstration

A. Van Gieson's Stain

1. Preparation of Weigert's Iron Hematoxylin

Solution A
- Harris hematoxylin—1 gm
- 95% ethanol—100 ml
  Allow the solution to ripen in bright day light for few days.

Solution B
- 30% ferric chloride—4 ml
- Conc. of HCl—1 ml
- Water—95 ml
  Before staining, mix equal volumes of freshly prepared solutions A and B.

2. Preparation of van Gieson's Stain
- Picric acid: 100 ml
- Acid fuscin: 100 ml
  These 2 solutions are mixed in the ratio of 5:1, hence van Gieson's stain is also called "Picrofuscin".

Steps for staining
1. Bring the sections to the water
2. Treat the sections with Weigert's iron hematoxylin for 20 minutes.
3. Differentiate in 1% acid alcohol
4. Blue in tap water
5. Treat the sections with van Gieson's stain for 3 minutes.
6. Clear in xylene
7. Mount with DPX

Results
- Nuclei: Blue/black
- Collagen: Red
- Smooth muscle and RBCs: Yellow

Note: van Gieson acts as a counterstain for Verhoeff's stain, von Kossa stain.

B. Masson's Trichrome Stain (MTS)

Solutions required.

A. Bouin's Solution

Ideal fixative for MTS.

B. Weigert's Iron Hematoxylin

Solution A
- Harris hematoxylin—1 gm
- 95% ethanol—100 ml
  Allow the solution to ripen in bright day light for few days.

Solution B
- 30% ferric chloride—4 ml
- Conc. of HCl—1 ml
- Water—95 ml
  Before staining, mix equal volumes of freshly prepared solutions A and B

C. Biebrich Scarlet Acid Fuscin Solution
- 1% aqueous Biebrich Scarlet—90 ml
- 1% aqueous acid fuscin—9 ml
- Glacial acetic acid: 1 ml

D. *Phosphomolybdic Acid–Phosphotungstic Acid (PMA-PTA) Solution*

- PMA—5 gm
- PTA—5 gm
- Distilled water—200 ml

E. *Light Green Solution*

- Light green yellowish—2 gm
- Water—98 ml
- Glacial acetic acid—2 ml

F. *1% Glacial Acetic Acid*

- Glacial acetic acid—1 ml
- Water—99 ml

Procedure

1. Deparaffinize and bring the sections to water
2. Treat sections with Bouin's solution for 1 hour at 56°C.
3. Wash with water thoroughly till the yellow color disappears.
4. Treat with Weigert's iron hematoxylin solution for 10 minutes.
5. Treat the sections with Biebrich Scarlet acid fuscin solution for 2 minutes.
6. Wash with water for 10 minutes
7. Treat the sections with PMA-PTA solution for 5 minutes.
8. Rinse with water
9. Treat the sections with light green stock solution for 5 minutes.
10. Treat the sections with glacial acetic acid for 1 minute.
11. Dehydrate in alcohol
12. Xylene
13. Mount in DPX

Results

- Nuclei: Blue black
- Collagen: Blue
- Muscle, keratin: Red

C. VGE Stain (for Elastic Fiber)

Reagents

1. *Verhoeff's hematoxylin (working solution)*
a. 5% alcoholic hematoxylin—20 ml
b. 10% ferric chloride—8 ml
c. Verhoeff's iodine—8 ml

Preparation

Take 10 ml of 5% alcoholic hematoxylin in a flask.

- Add 4 ml of 10% ferric chloride
- Mix well, than filter it
- Add 4 ml of Verhoeff's iodine

2. *Verhoeff's iodine*
a. Potassium iodide—4 gm
b. Iodine—2 gm
c. Distilled water—100 ml
   Mix well by grinding.

3. *2% ferric chloride*
a. Anhydrous ferric chloride—2 gm
b. Distilled water—100 ml

4. *van Gieson stain*
a. 1% aqueous acid fuscin—5 ml
b. Saturated aqueous picric acid—100 ml.

Procedure

1. Dewax the sections and bring to the water
2. Verhoeff's hematoxylin (working solution) for 10–15 minutes.
3. Wash with running tap water
4. Differentiate with 2% ferric chloride (1–2 minutes) microscopically.
5. At desired stage, stop the differentiation by quick dip in distilled water.
6. Counterstain with van Gieson stain for 1 minute.
7. Ethyl alcohol + few drops of saturated picric acid for 2–3 minutes.
8. Dry the sections and mount with DPX.

Results

- Elastic fiber—black color
- Nucleus—blue color
- Collagen—red color
- Muscle—yellow color

Tissue Processing

This chapter covers the following important topics:
a. Steps involved in tissue processing
b. Description of paraffin and its additives
c. Embedding technique
d. Decalcification

Aim of Tissue Processing

This involves a series of steps, which are designed to remove extractable water from the tissue, replacing it with a supporting medium that provides sufficient rigidity to enable sectioning of the tissue without the tissue being damaged or distorted.

Steps involved in tissue processing
1. Fixation
2. Dehydration
3. Clearing
4. Impregnation
5. Embedding
6. Cutting and staining
7. Section adhesion
8. Mountants

Salient Features

1. *Fixation* already discussed before in the other chapter of this book.
2. *Dehydration*
   - It is done for removal of unbound water and aqueous fixative from the tissue component.
   - Paraffin wax (in the coming steps) is not miscible with water and hence removal of water from the tissue is essential.
   - Dehydrating agent used should be 10 times the volume of tissue being dehydrated.
   - Examples of dehydrating agents: Ethyl alcohol, methanol, isopropyl alcohol, acetone, butyl alcohol and dioxane.

Note
   - Graded concentration of alcohol should be used starting from 70% followed by 95% and 100% solution.
   - Copper sulphate is placed at the bottom of a dehydrating bottle, which is covered with filter paper to prevent staining of the tissue, copper sulphate removes water from both alcohol and from the tissues.
   - In presence of water, copper sulphate changes its color from white to blue.

3. *Clearing*
   - Clearing agent acts as an intermediate between the dehydration and impregnation solutions.
   - Agent should be easily miscible within the solution.

Examples: Xylene, toluene, chloroform, methyl benzoate.

Properties of clearing agent
- Rapid removal of dehydrating agent
- Minimal tissue damage
- Ease of removal by melted wax (used in next step of tissue processing).

Procedure
- After dehydration, tissue is transferred into a clearing agent.
- Volume of the clearing agent should be 30–40 times the volume of the specimen.
- At least two changes should be given in a reagent like xylene.
- Small pieces of tissues get cleared in ½–1 hour.
- Biopsy specimen of 5 mm thickness takes—2 to 4 hours.

4. *Impregnation*
- The process of diffusion or infiltration of wax into the tissues is called impregnation.
- After clearing, the tissues are placed in paraffin wax in an embedding oven for infiltration and impregnation.
- Clearing agent is eliminated from the tissue by diffusion and molten wax is infiltrated.

Paraffin Wax
- It is routinely used as the impregnating and embedding media universally.
- Microcrystalline wax is a compound of high molecular weight having a melting point as high as 90°C.

Paraffin wax and its additives
Purpose
- Increases the hardness of the wax to cut thin sections at higher temperature.
- Increases the hardness to give support while sectioning harder tissues.
- Alter the crystalline structure of wax for better sectioning.
 Additives used are: Ceresin, beeswax

Types of paraffin
a. Liquid paraffin wax
b. Soft yellow paraffin wax
c. Soft white paraffin wax:
   - Commonly used in histology labs
   - It has a melting point of 56–64°
   - Available as a sheet, block or pellet forms
   - Volume of the wax should be used 25 times the volume of the tissue

5. *Embedding* (Figs 41.1 to 41.6)
- Process in which the tissue is enclosed in a mass of embedding medium using a mould.
- *Media:* Paraffin wax, celloidin, synthetic resins, gelatin.
- *Moulds:* Leukhardt L-shaped metal pieces, ice trays, paper boats, tissue-Tek system base moulds.

6. *Microtomy:* Already discussed in the other chapter of this book.

7. *Section adhesion*
Following adhesive agents can be used:
- Mayer's egg albumin

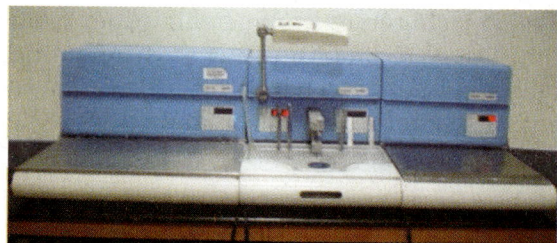

Fig. 41.1: Tissue-Tek system

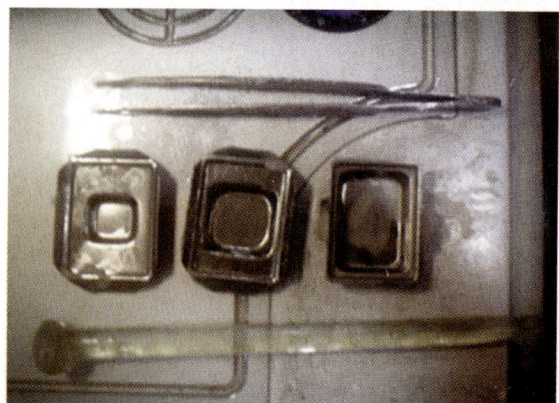

Fig. 41.2: Stainless steel base mold

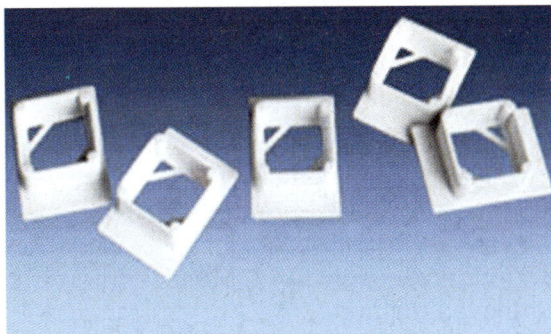

Fig. 41.3: Plastic rings

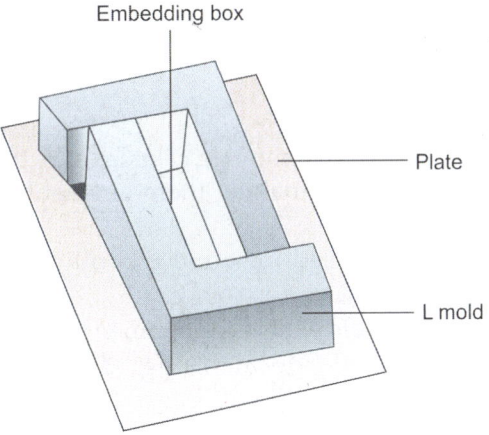

Fig. 41.6: Leukhardt's L-shaped mould

- Poly-L-lysine
- APTES (3-aminopropyltriethoxysilane)
- Albumin, gelatin and resins

8. *Mountants*
   - *Use:* To maintain high refractive index for microscopy and protect the sections during storage.
   - *Most commonly used mountant:* Kirkpatrick and Lendrum's DPX.

Automated tissue processor (Fig. 41.7):
- Processor in which station transfers (from one to another) of the tissue cassettes are done by using electro-mechanical mechanism.
- Programmable 24-hour clock

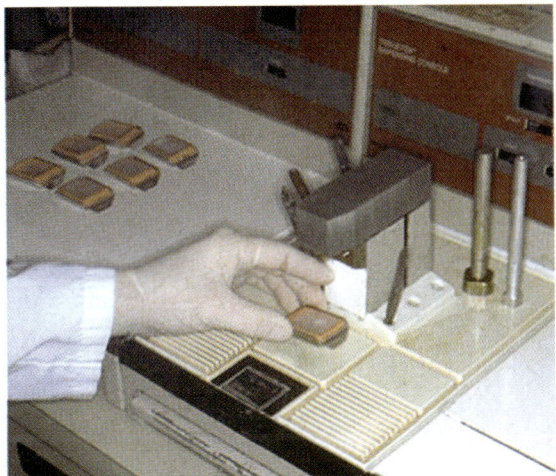

Fig. 41.4: Wax is being poured

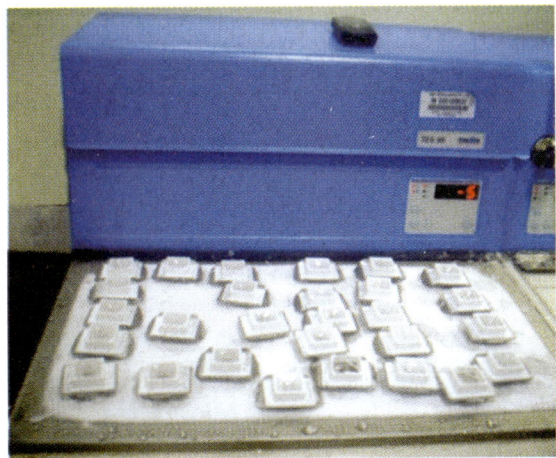

Fig. 41.5: Cold plate of embedding station

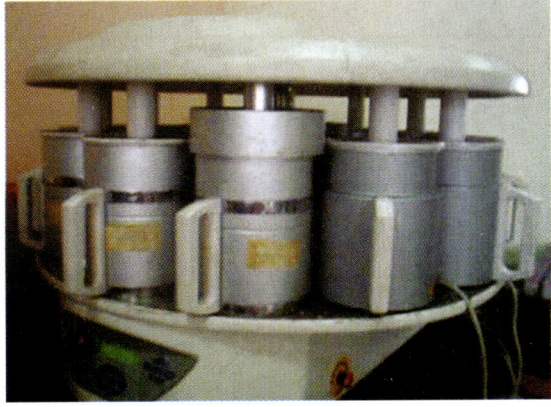

Fig. 41.7: Automated tissue processor

- 2 liters capacity glass breakers
- Thermostatically controlled wax bath

Decalcification

- The process of removing calcium salts from the tissue and making them amenable for sectioning.
- Method is used for bone and other hard tissues.
- Tissue should not exceed 5 mm in thickness.
- Volume of decalcifying fluid—50–100 times of the tissue.

Criteria fulfilling satisfactory decalcification
- Complete removal of calcium salts
- Lack of distortion of the cells and connective tissue.

Methods of decalcification
- Acid decalcification
- Ion exchange resins
- Electrical ionization
- Chelating methods
- Surface decalcification

Acid decalcification: Most commonly employed method

Decalcifying fluids
a. Strong acids (nitric acid, HCl, sulfuric acid)
b. Weak acids (formic acid, picric acid, acetic acid)

Note: Nitric acid and formic acid are most commonly used.

Section III

Histopathology and Cytology

Automation in Cytology

Goals to Achieve

- To produce faster and better results
- To reduce the time needed to perform the tests.
- Proper new techniques, which should be better in comparison to the original techniques.
- Large number of samples can be run simultaneously.
- Reducing the operator exposure to potential hazardous biological material.

Automation Devices

- Specimen collection and preparation devices.
- Manual screening devices.
- Automated screening devices.

a. Specimen Collection and Preparation Devices

- Earlier methods include the use of conventional smears preparation for cervical cytology.
- But, recently, this is being replaced by Thin Prep techniques.
- Thin Prep techniques include sample being thoroughly mixed with a fixative.
- Fixatives should lyse RBCs, mucus, large clumps of cells and allow easy transportation of the sample obtained to laboratory centers.
- Sample is directly obtained to slides from fixative solution and air-drying artifectual changes are minimal.

b. Manual Screening Devices

- Automated machines available can mark the specific portion of the slides.
- Only these portions of the slides will be reviewed by the Cytopathologist.
- This can save time in large laboratories
- Also, when the slide is examined, attached computer monitor can calculate the percentage fields examined by the cytopathologist.

c. Automated Screening Devices

- Computer software derived screening of the slides
- Instruments screen the slides and categorize them into "no further review slides or review required slides"
- "No further review slides" need not be examined by pathologist and these can be reported as negative
- "Review required slides" require screening by a pathologist.

Automation in Histopathology

What is the Need for Automation?

- Allows proper handling of the specimens in lab
- Reduces turnaround time
- Improves laboratory safety
- Reduces contamination
- Reduces cost
- Providing services of special stains, bio-markers, etc.

Is Automation Possible in Histopathology Lab?

Yes, it is possible. Except in grossing, which cannot be automated, automation plays a role in cassetting, embedding, microtomy, staining and coverslipping.

Benefits of Automation

1. *Faster Turnaround Times*

- Can make a lab more competitive and more patient-friendly with faster dispatch of tissue biopsies.
- Turnaround times with help of automation can be reduced from more than two days to less than one day.

2. *Reduced Contamination*

- Tissue fragments from one slide can be found on another slide.
- This is going to increase the time for processing for that particular case and can even result in erroneous reports.
- Automated devices can reduce the risk for contamination as it reduces human interaction with the tissue.

3. *Safety*

- Laboratory staff are in continuous exposure to the solvents like xylene.
- Xylene can lead to irritation of the skin, eyes, nose, throat, lungs or in longer duration can affect kidneys, heart, lungs, nervous system.
- Automated tissue processor has significantly reduced this hazard of exposure.
- Microtome induced hand injuries, can be significantly reduced, due to the advent of automation.
- Automation also reduces the stress on laboratory personnel.

Electron Microscopy

Introduction to Electron Microscope

- Uses electrons to illuminate a specimen and create an enlarged image.
- Have much greater resolving power than light microscope and can obtain higher magnifications.
- Can provide high magnification to the tissues, so that tissue details can be studied.
- Images can be stored by using digital cameras.

Types

a. *Transmission electron microscope*

Principles (Fig. 44.1)

- A beam of electrons is focused on a sample
- The electrons pass through the sample to form an image on a fluorescent screen.

b. *Scanning electron microscope*

Principles (Fig. 44.2):

- A beam of electrons is focused on the surface of a sample.
- Secondary electrons are emitted from the sample surface.
- A detector is used to form an image from the secondary electrons.

Other types of electron microscope:

c. *Reflection electron microscope*

d. *Scanning transmission electron microscope*

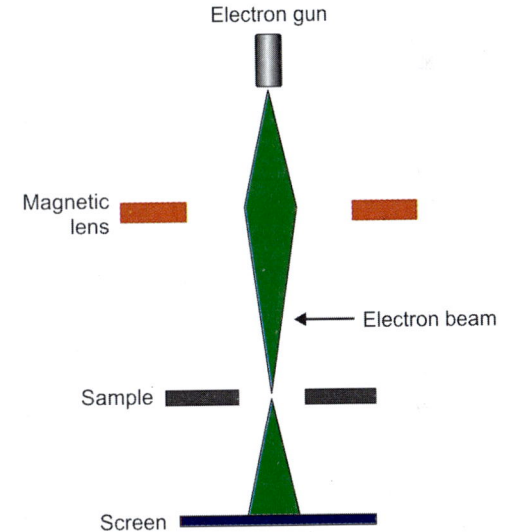

Fig. 44.1: Principle of transmission electron microscope

Uses of Electron Microscopy

1. Mainly in research related work
2. Renal and skin biopsy interpretation
3. To visualize the structure of cell, micro-organisms, biopsy samples, metals, crystals.

Sample Preparation

Important points of how a tissue biopsy for electron microscopy should be dealt:

- *Chemical fixation* by cross-linking of proteins by using formaldehyde, glutaraldehyde, osmium tetraoxide.

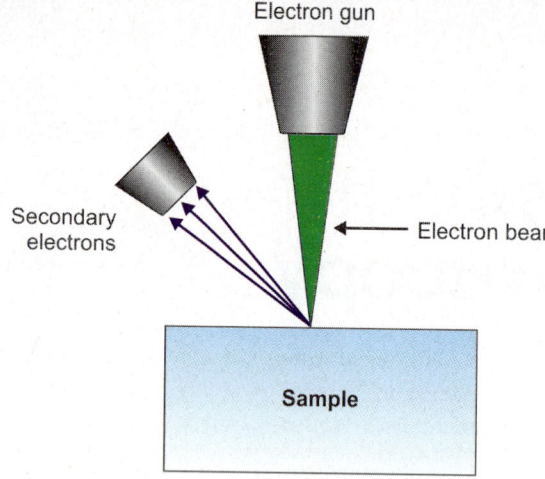

Fig. 44.2: Principle of scanning electron microscope

- *Dehydration:* Replacement of water with acetone or ethanol.
- *Embedding:* After dehydration, tissue is embedded in resin, following which ultrathin sections are taken.
- *Sectioning:* Disposable glass knives or an ultramicrotome with a diamond knife is used to take ultrathin sections of 60–90 nm thick.
- These sections are stained using heavy metals such as lead, uranium or tungsten and are visualized under microscope.

Disadvantages of Electron Microscope

- Expensive to build and maintain
- Requires special buildings to keep as the device requires high resolution.

Photography and Gross Microphotography

- Today is a world of digital imaging
- Digital imaging has changed the outlook of surgical pathology.
- Digital images of the gross specimens and the microscopic slides can be shared throughout the world, for educational purposes.
- Digital images are now being included in reports of the patients.
- It helps in documentation in support of making the diagnosis.
- Digital photography has created a vast interest amongst pathologists in the fields of telepathology/telemicroscopy.
- Live image display with the help of digital cameras can be introduced to the people in live meetings, and this branch has been given a name of robotic telepathology.
- Automated digital cameras are now being installed at grossing stations, for capturing the macroscopic images of the gross samples.
- Digital images enhance the quality and accuracy of pathology reports.
- Slide digitization can change the way of examination of tissue sections and also its storage.
- Reduction in the costs of this technology in near-future, will enable digital imaging in surgical pathology laboratories an essential consideration.

Grossing and Specimen Management

1. Surgical pathology is a branch of pathology, which deals with grossing of surgical specimens.

2. As the surgical specimen is received in the histopathology laboratory, it is given an identification number, which will be unique to that particular specimen and that number will be kept in records of the laboratory for lifetime.

3. Laboratory personal has to ensure that the specimen received should have adequate formalin and the requisition form details should include name, age, sex, clinical diagnosis and relevant history of the patient, before acceptance of the specimen.

4. After this the specimen is taken to the grossing station and if adequate fixation of the tissue is achieved, the processing of the tissue will start.

5. In cases of large gross specimens, the specimen should be appropriately cut with help of the large blade and new formalin should be added, amount of which should be ten times the size of the specimen.

6. For large specimens like colon, adequate size of bucket should be used.

7. After fixation, the specimen should be grossed according to the protocol followed in that particular institution.

8. It is the responsibility of the pathologist, to make sure that the specimen should not be distorted or mutilated in any way, while taking appropriate tissue sections from the specimen.

9. Small biopsies should be processed as a whole.

10. While grossing, the size of the specimen, its margins, any abnormalities noted on gross examination should be described.

11. If any tumor mass is detected, on cut surface of the specimen, it should be described in terms of its diameter, extension, margins, extent up to the deeper layers of the mucosa, its cut surface and appearance should be recorded.

12. If the specimen is a rare specimen, it can be stored for academic interest.

13. After, the report is dispatched; the specimen should be discarded according to the laboratory protocol.

14. Usually small specimens and non-malignant specimens are discarded after three weeks of dispatching the report.

15. In case of malignant specimens, they need to be stored for longer duration, if institution has academic interest.

16. For grossing of large specimens, proper guidelines should be made for grossing as well as for microscopic reporting.

Management of Cytological Specimen

Management of cytological specimen includes
- Receiving of the specimen and request form
- Preparation of the slides for microscopic examination.
- Staining, screening and reporting the slides

All these processes are subject to quality control and quality assurance measures.

Receiving of the Specimen and Request Form
- It is the duty of laboratory personnel to check the details written on the specimen and form, whether these details are matching or not.
- Specimen and form must have at least three-patient identifiers (which include name, surname, date of birth, patients hospital registration number).
- Laboratory reference number is assigned to the sample.
- Patient hospital number and sample (laboratory) reference number are noted in a register or in a computerized system.

Preparation of Slides

Slides are prepared and these are either stained with Giemsa stain, hematoxylin and eosin stain, Pap stain.

Note: Details about all these stains can be read from the respective sections of other chapters of this book.

Screening and Reporting of Slides
- After, the slides are ready, Cytopathologist evaluates the slides.
- If the material is inadequate for opinion, this information is provided in the report and is signed out and a reaspirate or a fresh sample is asked for in the report.
- If the material is adequate for reporting, the report with the diagnosis, based on the findings are signed off, with an appropriate advise to the physician, if and when required.
- These reports before being dispatched are entered in a register for documentation or in a computer-based software.
- Report can be handed over to the patient or can be put up in a computer software for the physician to look into it.

Note: Also go through the chapter of quality control in cytology of this book.

Sources, Types of Cytological and Histopathological Specimens

Types of Material Obtained in Histopathological Laboratory

a. *Incisional tissue biopsy:* A small piece of lesion or tumor which in sent for the diagnosis before final removal of the lesion or tumor.

b. *Excisional biopsy:* If the whole of the tumor or lesion is sent for examination and diagnosis to the pathologist.

c. Tissues from the autopsy are sent for the study of disease and its course.

Most common source of biopsy received in a laboratory includes: Endometrial biopsies, skin biopsy, lymph node biopsy, thyroid specimens, breast specimens, liver biopsy, CNS biopsy, kidney biopsy or specimens, prostatic biopsy, soft tissue specimens, bone specimens, and bone marrow biopsy.

Types and Sources of Cytological Specimens

a. Fine needle aspiration cytology smears made from the swellings present over the body.

b. *Gastrointestinal washings:* Colonic brushings and washings, duodenal and gastric washings, esophageal washings, rectal washings.

c. Lung/bronchial aspirate and washings [Bronchio-alveolar lavage (BAL) fluid]

d. Pleural, pericardial and ascitic fluid studies

e. Sputum studies

f. Urine cytology

g. CSF cytology

h. Ectocervical and endocervical brushings, which are processed by performing a Pap stain.

Section IV

Laboratory Management

Chapters

Biomedical Waste (BMW) Management

How is the Hospital Waste Classified?

It is being classified on the basis of the waste being disposed to a particular bag designed for it.

Below mentioned criteria are in accordance to the biomedical waste management rules.

A. Following Waste should be Discarded in Yellow Containers

Type of waste	Treatment and disposal
Human anatomical waste: Human tissues, organs, body parts, fetus	Incineration, plasma pyrolysis, deep burial
Animal anatomical waste: Animal carcasses, body parts, organs, tissues and waste generated from animals during experiments	Incineration, plasma pyrolysis, deep burial
Soiled waste: Items contaminated with blood, body fluids like dressings, plaster casts, cotton swabs, bags, discarded blood and blood components	Incineration, plasma pyrolysis, deep burial
Expired or discarded medicines: Pharmaceutical waste like antibiotics, cytotoxic drugs	To be returned back to the manufacturer, or incineration or plasma pyrolysis at 1200°C
Chemical waste: Chemical used in production of biological and used or discarded disinfectants	Incineration, plasma pyrolysis, encapsulation in hazardous waste treatment, storage and disposal facility
Chemical liquid waste used or discarded disinfectants, formalin infected secretions, aspirated body fluids, liquids from laboratories and floor washing, cleaning and house-keeping activities	After resource recovery, the chemical liquid waste shall be pre-treated before mixing with other waste water
Discarded linen, mattresses, beddings contaminated with blood or body fluids	Incineration, plasma pyrolysis, energy recovery
Other laboratory waste: Blood bags, laboratory culture, specimens of microorganisms, live or attenuated vaccines, human and animal cell cultures used in research, industrial laboratories	Pre-treat to sterilize non-chlorinated chemicals as per NACO or WHO guidelines thereafter for incineration

Note: Pyrolysis means decomposition brought about by high temperatures.

B. Following Waste should be Discarded in Red Containers

Type of waste	Treatment and disposal
Contaminated waste (recyclable): Waste generated from disposable items such as tubing, bottles, intravenous tubes, catheters, urine bags, syringes without needles and vacutainers with their needles cut and gloves.	Autoclaving or microwaving/hydroclaving followed by shredding or mutilation or combination of sterilization and shredding

C. Following Waste should be Discarded in Blue Boxes (Cardboard Boxes with Blue-colored Markings)

Type of waste	Treatment and disposal
Glassware: Broken or discarded glassware and contaminated glass including medicine vials and ampoules except those contaminated with cytotoxic waste	Disinfection after cleaning with detergent and sodium hypochlorite or through autoclaving, hydroclaving and then sent for recycling

D. Following Waste should go in White Containers (Translucent)

Type of waste	Treatment and disposal
Waste sharps including metals: Needles, syringes with fixed needles, scalpels, blades, or any other contaminated object that may cause cuts and punctures	Autoclaving or dry heat sterilization followed by shredding or mutilation or encapsulation in metal container or cement concrete; combination of shredding-cum-autoclaving and sent for final disposal to iron foundries or designated concrete waste sharp pit

E. Following Waste should be Discarded in Black Containers

General wastes like non-infected plastics, cardboard, packaging material, paper.

Note: Defaulters are liable to be prosecuted/fined up to Rs. one lakh and 5 years of imprisonment.

Handling of BMW

i. Wear appropriate gloves, clothing cover, safety glasses while handling non-inactivated waste.
   a. Use universal precautions—assume all BMW as infectious.
   b. Transport waste in leakproof containers.
   c. Know how to handle spills.
ii. Documentation of all the bags stored, transported and disposed, shall be carried out by authorized personnel.

BMW Storage

BMW must be stored in an area away from general traffic and accessible only to authorized personnel.

Storage area must be:
- Labeled with a biohazard sticker
- Secure (locked/non-accessible)
- Easily cleanable and tidy
- Packages must be labeled as biomedical waste with the biohazard symbol, name, location, phone and date.
- Then transport it to outdoor containers removed for disposal by a designated waste disposal authority.

Note: Also go through the chapter of methods of disposal of pathological waste.

Hospital Organization and Operations

Hospital Organization (Figs 50.1 and 50.2)

An organization conveys information related to various posts with associated responsibilities, their hierarchical arrangement and communication pattern in the organization.

Hospital Operations

- Function and role of the hospital depends on the population, it caters to as well as the existing healthcare system in the population

- Primary function of hospital is treatment of patient either on emergency, outpatient or inpatient basis.

- Hospital also functions as centers of preventive health, medical education and research.

- Hospitals also have a role in economy of the locality as hospitals are one of the major sources of employment.

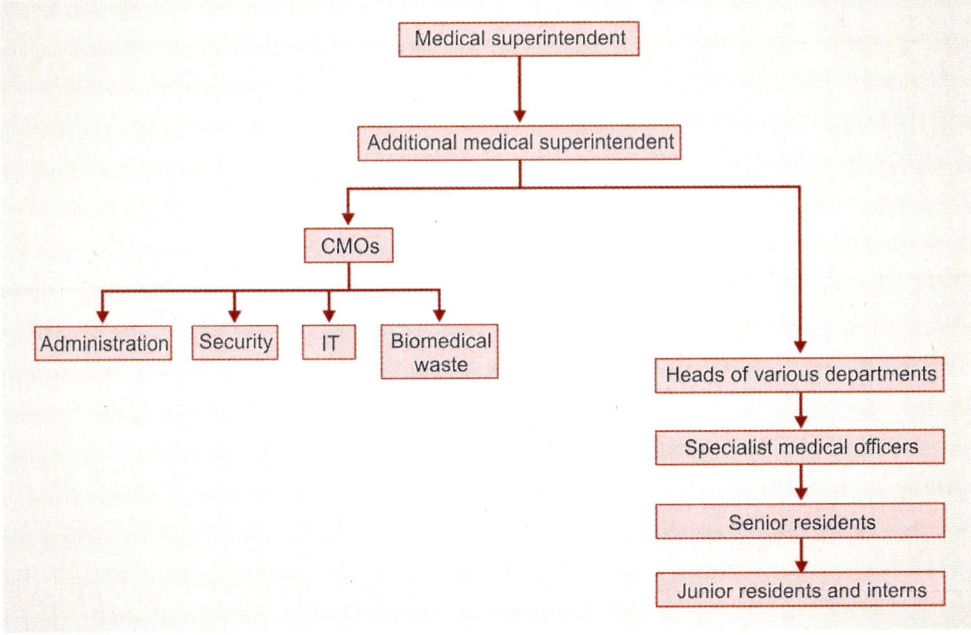

Fig. 50.1: Organization of medical staff in hospital (CMO—casualty medical officer, IT—information technology)

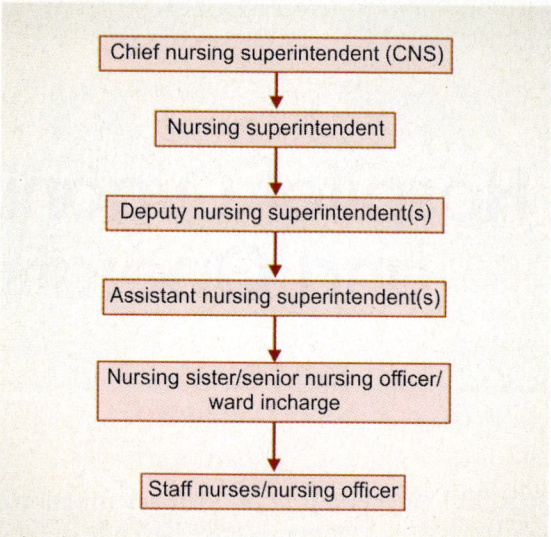

Fig. 50.2: Organization of nursing staff in hospital

Internal Quality Control Involving Quantitative Results

- Quantitative results are obtained in hematology and biochemistry sections.
- Internal quality control of quantitative results can be done by:
  1. Measurements done on control material
  2. Repeated measurements on the routine specimens
  3. Statistical analysis of the data obtained daily from analyzers.
  4. Analysis of normal (AoN)

For Control Material

- Control material is analyzed alongside the batch of routine specimens.
- Commercially prepared control materials have their mean and standard deviation specified.
- Each laboratory should establish its laboratory mean and laboratory standard deviation by running the control.
- The results of control material from each batch are plotted on Levey-Jennings chart.
- The chart has horizontal lines, which correspond to the mean, +1SD, +2SD, +3SD, –1SD, –2SD, –3SD.
- For interpretation of charts certain rules are used, known as Westgard rules (Westgard, 1981).

Westgard Rules (Fig. 51.1)

- Ideally in a clinical laboratory 3 levels of control are run (low, normal, and high).
- At least two levels of control are run in each batch.
- When the results are out of control, root-cause analysis of the problem is done and after correction of problem, the batch in question is rerun with control material.

Westgard Rules

1_{2S} rule
1_{3S} rule
2_{2S} rule
R_{4S} rule
4_{1S} rule
10_X rule

1_{2S} *rule:* When one control value is outside 2SD. It is a warning rule.

1_{3S} *rule:* When one control value is outside 3SD. It is a rejection rule.

2_{2S} *rule:* When two consecutive control values are outside 2SD or both levels of control are outside 2SD. It is a rejection rule.

R_{4S} *rule:* The difference between two control values is more than or equal to 4 times SD. It is a rejection rule.

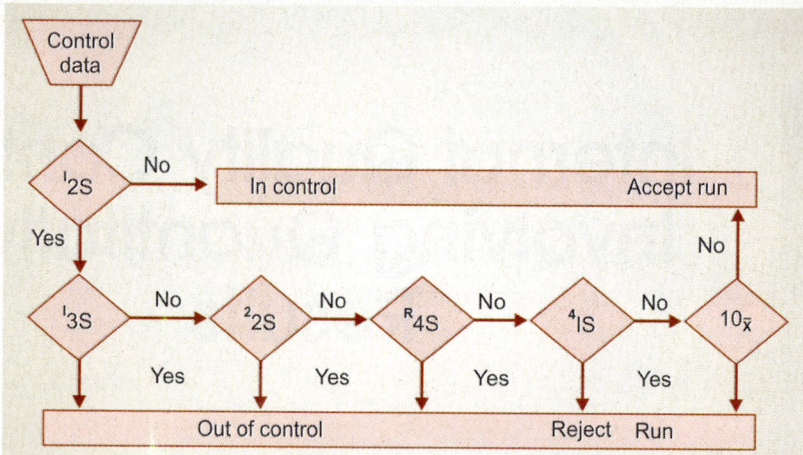

Fig. 51.1: Algorithm for application of Westgard rules

4_{1S} *rule:* When 4 consecutive control measurements exceed the same mean plus 1s or the same mean minus 1S control limit. It is a rejection rule.

10_X *rule:* When 10 consecutive control measurements fall on one side of the mean. It is a rejection rule.

Inventories

Inventory is defined as stock or store of goods.

What is Inventory Management?

- Planning and controlling of inventory from raw material stage to delivery of product/ service to the customer.
- Divided into: (1) Aggregate inventory management, (2) item inventory management.

1. Aggregate Inventory Management

Deals with the classification, need, and cost associated with inventory

A. Classification:
  - Raw materials
  - Work in process (WIP)
  - Finished goods
  - Distribution inventories
  - Maintenance, repair and operational supplies (MRO)

B. Need for inventories: Depends on the demand for the products

C. Objectives for inventories:
  - Maximum customer service
  - Low cost
  - Minimum investment

2. Item Inventory Management

Following questions must be answered for proper item inventory management.

A. *How important a particular inventory is?* Implies that each item should receive a weighed treatment corresponding to its class.

Can be understood by ABC approach, in which the items are rated from A to C:
- A items consist of the goods of which the annual consumption value is the highest.
- B items consist of the goods with medium consumption value
- C items consist of the goods with the lowest consumption value.

Control based on ABC classification
- *A items (high priority):* Tight control including complete accurate records, regular and frequent review by the management, frequent review of demand forecasts, and close follow-up and expediting to reduce lead time.
- *B items (medium priority):* Normal controls with good records, regular attention and normal processing.
- *C items (lowest priority)* can keep extra one unit in hand.

B. *When should a purchase order be placed?*
Following system should be used:
- Order point system
- Periodic review system
- Material requirement planning

C. *How much quantity should be ordered at a time?*
It is important to order, a fixed quantity, which is known as "economic order quantity (EOQ)".

Job Analysis

Human resource management should understand the strategic plans of the business as well as job descriptions and job specifications.

Job description: The content (duties and responsibilities) plus context (physical and personnel environment) of the job.

Job specifications: The knowledge, skills and abilities required to perform the job.

Job description and job specifications are the output of job analysis.

Steps of a Job Analysis Process

Step 1 Describe the purpose of job analysis
Step 2 Select the required job from organization chart
Step 3 Gathering of data
Step 4 Writing the results (job description + job specifications)

Various Methods for Gathering of Data for Job Analysis

a. *Questionnaires:* A questionnaire is given to job holders who can answer the questions at their convenient time. However, the results are dependent on recollecting powers and communicating abilities of job holders.

b. *Interviews* in one to one interview unlike the questionnaire method, interviewer can explain the questions. However, there are chances of interviewer's bias.

c. *Observations:* Routine and repetitive jobs can be easily analyzed by observing the job holders. However, there are chances of observer bias and this method is unsuitable for knowledge-based job.

d. *Participant's diary/ law:* In this, job holder fills up the diary as and when he or she performs the task. However, there are chances of job holder's bias as he/she may not enter the task, which he/she seem unimportant.

Recent Advance

- Nowadays, there is no need to correlate the formal job descriptions and specifications, as individuals can be hired on the basis of required competency.
- Competency is identified as an attribute, which an employee must possess in order to perform related jobs.

Management Review Meetings

Introduction

- Management review meetings are done to monitor and review the goals set for a particular year.
- It ensures improvement of the management system.
- Goals are being set, monitored and reviewed by the laboratory manager.

Objectives

Following points need to be focused upon:
- Information arising from internal audits
- Major changes in operation of the laboratory
- Correct and timely implementation of the quality management system.
- Feedback (complaints, satisfaction surveys, etc.) from staff and customers.
- Identification of the new opportunities for improvement.
- Allocation of resources for follow-up actions.

Inputs of a Review

Following can serve as input for the management review:

- Positives and negatives originating from the last management review.
- Achievement of goals set in the quality year plan.
- Result of the selection and assessment of suppliers to the laboratory.
- Assessment of the turnaround times
- Competence of personnel and their training needs
- Report of external quality assessments
- Report of internal and external quality audits and their follow-up.
- Quarterly quality reports
- Complaint forms.

Final Conclusion

Findings of the management review are recorded in the management review report. This report describes:
- Decisions made
- Description of discussion behind the decisions made.
- Follow-up actions
- Conclusions.

55

Maintenance of Laboratory Refrigerators, Freezers and Other Equipment

- Laboratory refrigerator should never be used for storage of edibles and drinks.
- Laboratory refrigerator is used for preservation of samples, prior to the analysis.
- No sample should be kept exposed, but should be sealed in plastic.
- Light sensitive samples require storage in dark pouches or amber-colored vials.
- Labels should be properly affixed and covered with a transparent film.
- Store samples, chemicals in appropriate temperature zones, according to their temperature requirements.
- Clean the cabinets and shelves only after disconnecting the power at least on weekly basis.
- Requires daily calibration and maintenance of calibration records.
- A calibrated thermometer is placed in a beaker containing silicone oil in different drawers and freezers. The door is closed and after stabilizing for 15 minutes, temperature readings are recorded. The temperature in cabinets should range from 2° to 8°C.
- The temperature in deep freezers should range between –10° and –20°C.
- If the temperature is still not within the acceptable range and adjusting the thermostat has not solved the problem, move the contents of the refrigerator to another refrigerator and contact an engineer.
- Dispose of materials which could have been damaged. Record corrective actions on the temperature chart.
- Interior of the refrigerator should be decontaminated periodically.
- Exterior of the refrigerator should be cleaned, when necessary with a damp cloth and mild soap.

MAINTENANCE OF TISSUE EMBEDDING SYSTEM

A. Removal of Wax

- Disconnect instrument from mains power supply when cleaning.
- Use only plastic or wooden implements to scrape off wax.
- Use only minimal quantities of solvent on an absorbent cloth.
- Also the paraffin reservoir needed to be cleaned of wax by these methods.

B. For Base Molds Warming Oven

- Disconnect instrument from the mains power supply.
- Wipe the inside of the oven with a tissue moistened with a xylene substitute.
- Need to be cleaned once every two weeks.

C. Cold Plate

- Switch off the instrument and allow the cold plate to defrost
- Frequently wipe the cold spot with a cloth to absorb any condensation
- Condensation that forms on the cold plate, should be drained, through special channels on either side of the cold plate area into the drip tray below.

D. Work Stage

- The work stage has a slight gradient that directs excess molten wax towards the tissue holding tank.
- At the end of the operation, or more often if needed, wipe down the surface of the work stage with an absorbent cloth.
- Condensation that may form on the cold spot should not be allowed to enter the tissue holding tank.
- Frequently wipe the cold spot with a cloth to absorb any condensation.
- Perform these steps daily.

E. Paraffin Reservoir

- After use and normally when the wax level is low, empty the reservoir by continuous operation of the paraffin dispenser switch or foot switch. Collect molten wax in a suitable receptacle (hollow object).
- Depress the heating elements to switch off and remove residual wax with absorbent cloth.
- Remove the filter screen and clean the screen using a xylene substitute.
- Replace the filter screen and refill the paraffin reservoir with molten or palletized wax.
- Perform these steps every two to four weeks.

F. Tissue Holding Tank

- Switch off the heating elements and allow the paraffin in the tank to solidify. When the instrument is cool, press the heating elements button to turn the tissue holding tank on.
- After 15 minutes, the wax around the edges of the bath should melt and the remaining solidified wax can be removed as a block by lifting the drainage ledge.
- Switch off the instrument and disconnect from the mains. Residual wax in the tank may now be removed using an absorbent cloth.
- Once cleaned, refill with molten wax or palletized paraffin pellets, reconnect with mains and switch on.
- Perform these steps once or twice a week.

Parts (Fig. 55.1)

- Mold warmer, cassette bath, working surface warmer, forceps well.
- Cold plate: –5° to +5°C
- Large 3–5 liters capacity paraffin reservoir with adjustable temperature of 45–75°C.
- Forceps warmer, convenient drain for excess wax.

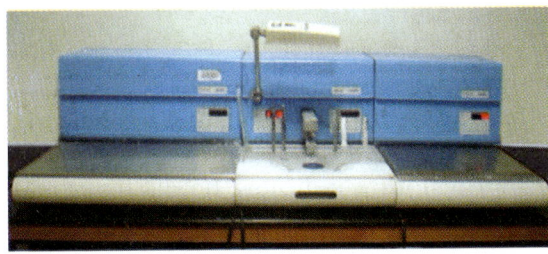

Fig. 55.1: Tissue embedding system

Material Safety Data Sheet (MSDS)

Document which provides the information on a product in relation to:

a. Health effects of exposure to the product
b. Hazardous effect in relation to the product storage, handling and use.
c. Measure to protect workers at risk of exposure.
d. Emergency procedures.

Content of MSDS

- *Hazardous ingredients:* Chemical names and concentrations, concerning the hazardous ingredients.
- *MSDS preparation information:* The name, address, telephone number and the date when MSDS was prepared.
- *Product information* identifies the product by the name on the supplier label, its chemical name, family and formula (including molecular weight).
- *Physical data* indicates, how it looks and how it will behave when it is used, stored, spilled and how it will react with other products indicated.

- *Reactivity data* implies, chemical stability of the product and its reactions to light, heat, moisture, shock.
- *Toxicology properties* include the harmful effects of the exposure, how the product is likely to enter the body, and what effects it has on the organs of the body including both short-term (acute) and long-term (chronic).
- *Preventive measures* include the instruction for the safe use, handling and storage of the product, personal protective equipment or the safety devices required.
- *First aid measures* include specific first aid measures related to the acute effects of exposure to the product.

Material safety data sheets (MSDS) or other chemical hazard information is available from chemical manufacturers and or suppliers.

They should be accessible in laboratories, where these chemicals are used, e.g. as part of a safety or operations manual.

Medical Ethics and their Role in Laboratory Medicine

Principle of Medical Ethics

"Doing good and not doing harm is the basic principle of medical ethics".

Since medical laboratory technology (MLT) affects patient care, general principles of medical ethics also apply to MLT practice.

Ethics in MLT practice can be discussed as follows

1. Collection of Information

- Adequate information needs to be obtained from the patient.
- Demographic information is required for sample identification, billing purpose and clinical interpretation of laboratory results.
- Patient should be aware of the information collection and the purpose for which it is collected.
- The information must be stored securely.
- Duration of information storage should be defined in laboratory policies.
- Overseas transmission of information may be restricted by law.

2. Collection of Specimen

- Before collection of any specimen, consent is necessary.
- Patient in a hospital bed should be given the opportunity to refuse.
- Consent might not be possible in emergency situations.
- Specimen collection should ensure sufficient privacy.

3. Special Procedures

- Special procedure like bone marrow examination or fine needle aspiration cytology or sampling for HIV testing requires informed and written consent.
- Pre-test counseling is done before sampling for HIV testing.

4. Reporting of Results

- Patient results are confidential and should be disclosed only to the patient or treating clinician.
- Language and format of the report should facilitate its correct interpretation and diagnosis.
- It is the responsibility of the laboratory to convey critical results as soon as they are available.

5. Retention of Medical Records/Specimen

- Duration of retention of medical records/specimens should be defined by the laboratory policy.
- NABL has also laid down guidelines for the same.

- Information must be safeguarded against loss/tempering and unauthorized access.

6. Financial Arrangement

- Implies financial understanding between the clinician and laboratory.
- Such a financial arrangement is harmful for the patient as well as the medical profession.

7. Research

- Laboratory plays an important role in the biomedical research.
- Hence, laboratory should ensure that institutional ethical clearance is in place, proper consent is taken, privacy and confidentiality is maintained throughout the research.

Principles of Laboratory Management

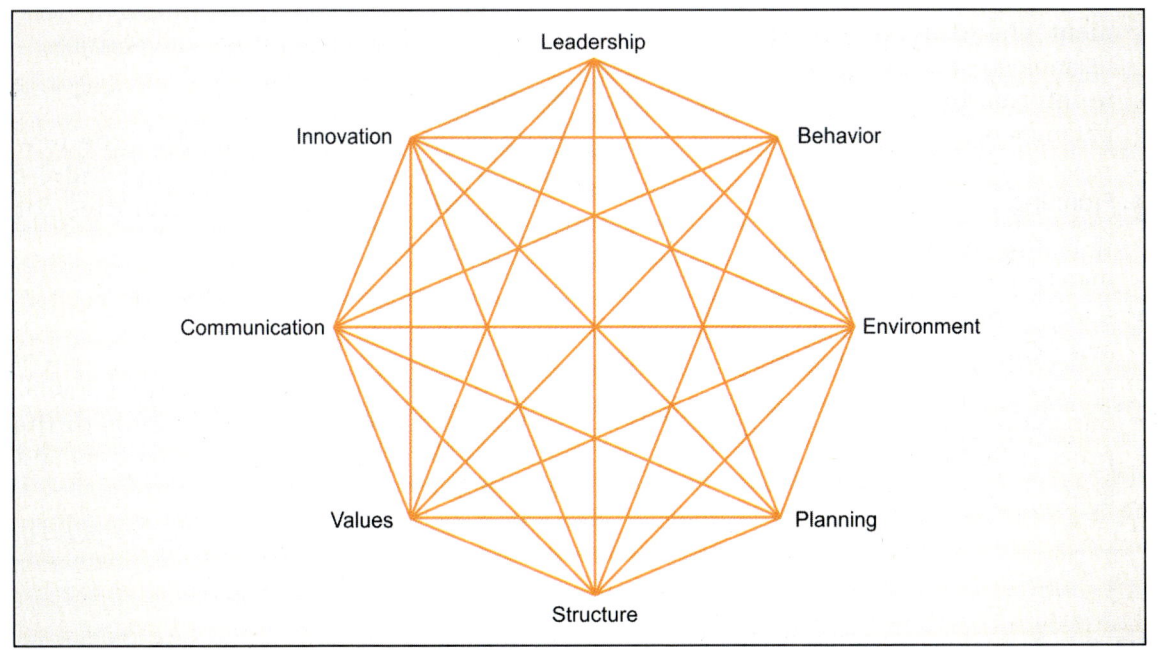

Fig. 58.1: Eight principles of laboratory management

Principles of laboratory management are demonstrated in Fig. 58.1 above. These are interrelated and all of them have equal importance.

Note: The interrelation of principles will produce quality laboratory services for patients, primary health care providers, and the laboratorians themselves.

Each principle can be characterized as follows.

1. Leadership

- Different from management
- Implies influenced by example and motivation
- Leadership quality is not necessarily inborn, but can be learned and honed.

2. Behavior

- Organization behavior is important for an individual to succeed and meet the organization needs.

- Most important attribute for organization behavior is understanding an individual psychology.

3. Environment

- Can be influenced by external and internal factors.
- *External environment:* One should be well verse with knowledge of the social, demographic, political, regulatory body, peer review issues with media and public relation issues.
- *Internal environment* includes institutional and workforce issues. Laboratorian environment changes are brought about by technology and testing methods, advances in information management, regulatory parameters and enforcement.

4. Planning

- It is the most important principle of management.
- Every laboratory should establish a mission and vision depending upon the customer needs.
- Successful planning implies implantation process that transforms ideal strategies, goals and objectives into reality.

5. Structure

Understanding of organizational configuration, including the history of their development.

6. Values

In every laboratory, there should be understanding of individual human rights, professional ethics, patient rights and employee rights.

7. Communication

- It should be designed for flow of data and information, either to the patient or colleagues.
- Various modes of communication can be computers, electronic and printing devices, telephones and one to one conversation.

8. Innovation

Includes the ability to introduce the new approaches, methods or devices to address old problems or new opportunities for improvement.

Note: Successful change requires leaders who are champions of innovation.

Effective interrelationship of the above eight principles will produce quality laboratory services that will satisfy the needs of the patients, primary healthcare providers and laboratorians themselves.

Quality Control

General Aspects

- Quality control is to keep a check on the result of measurement procedures.
- It is done in order to verify that all tests, being performed in a laboratory, are being done as per specifications.
- There are certain terms related to measurements, materials and methods with respect to quality control.

Components for Quality Control

Measurements	Materials	Methods
Standard deviation	Reference material	Reference method
Co-efficient of variance	Calibrator	Selected method
Accuracy	Control material	Working method
Precision		

Measurements

1. Standard Deviation (SD)

- Also known as root mean square deviation
- An absolute measure of dispersion
- Average deviation of values from the mean.

2. Co-efficient of Variance (CV)

- Measurement of the dispersion of data
- Useful to compare different groups (results of different analytics)

- It is given by the formula:

$$CV = \frac{SD \times 100}{Mean}$$

3. Accuracy

- Closeness of the result/value to that (value) which is considered to be true.
- Achieved by the use of reference material or calibrators.
- Can be achieved by participating in EQAS programs.

4. Precision

Closeness between the different values of data obtained under repeatability conditions.

Materials

1. *Reference material:* Serve to assign value to secondary standards/calibrators.
2. *Control*
   - For statistical control on measurement process.
   - Are used to measure precision.

Methods

1. *Reference methods*
   - Used in association with reference material to provide accurate and precise data for critical scientific purposes.
   - Used for validating selected methods

2. *Selected method*

Used for validating a routine working method.

3. *Routine working methods*

- Reliable method for routine use
- Modification of selected method, considering the economy of labor/material and ease of performance.

Classification

Quality control in a clinical laboratory can be divided into:

1. Internal quality control (IQC)
2. External quality assurance (EQA)

Differences between Internal Quality Control and External Quality Assurance

See below

Internal quality control	External quality assurance
It is internal to the institution	It is external to the institution
It is prospective in nature	It is retrospective in nature
It takes care of precision	It takes care of precision (if duplicate results are sent) and also accuracy indirectly

Quality Control in Cytology

Quality control in cytology is important to bring the measures that will improve the quality of cytology laboratory.

Each laboratory director should strictly adhere to the following regulations:

a. Correlate the cytological diagnosis with surgical and clinical findings of the patient.
b. Reevaluate those cases in which the cytological and histological or clinical history does not correlate.
c. Reviewing the records of previous cytological and histological examinations of each patient.
d. Prepare annual statistical correlation reports.
e. Maintain the data for number of cases with positive findings.
f. Retain the reports and slides in a readily accessible area for at least three years.
g. Encourage the technicians for participating in continuing medical education programs.
h. To bring about internal performance evaluation programs to demonstrate the competency and accuracy of technical personnel.

Reporting of Cytological Material

Report must include

1. Name of patient and the laboratory accession number.
2. Name of individual or facility to which the report is addressed.
3. Name and address of the laboratory
4. Following dates: Sample collection, sample received in the laboratory and report issued.
5. Cytological diagnosis
6. Identification of cytopathologist and cytotechnologist responsible for the report.

Other important points to be taken care of include:

• Laboratory should be clean, well lighted, adequately ventilated, and functionally arranged.
• Laboratory personnel must be protected against hazards (chemical, electric, fire, infections).
• Adequate number of binocular microscopes of good quality must be available.
• Specimens should be accepted and examined, if they are being sent by a registered medical physician.
• Laboratory should have a written criteria for rejecting specimens.
• Staining solutions and chemicals used in cytopathology laboratory should be labeled with the time of preparation, purchase, or both.
• Staining solutions should be filtered regularly to avoid the contamination and should be covered when not in use.
• Gynecological cytology should be reported using Bethesda system.

External Quality Assurance Programme

In cytopathology, unstained slides are distributed to the laboratories enrolled in the programme, from the main accredited laboratory, which is pursuing it.

Following parameters are noted for each participant:

i. Staining quality
ii. Mounting quality
iii. Labeling quality
iv. Description of microscopic findings
v. Final impression
vi. Special staining if performed.

Quality Assurance in Hematology

Aim of Quality Assurance

- Main aim of quality assurance is to ensure, whether the information produced by the laboratory is correct or not.
- Quality assurance includes the study of control charts, results produced, choice of methods used, training of personnel, handling of specimens and reporting results.

Three major activities of quality assurance

1. *Preventive activities*
   - These are done prior to the examination of the specimen or sample.
   - Help in establishing the systems, which help to maintain the accuracy in analytical testing (e.g. preventive maintenance and calibration of instruments, testing of media, orientation and training of personnel).
2. *Assessment:* To determine, whether the test systems are performing correctly (e.g. the use of standard and controls, maintenance of control charts).
3. *Corrective measures:* Measure taken, after an error is detected, to correct the system (e.g. equipment troubleshooting, recalibration of instruments).

Objective of Quality Assurance Programme

a. *Precision*
   - Reproducibility of results, whether accurate or inaccurate within a defined frame time (e.g. within the same day, from week to week, etc.).
   - It is controlled by replicate tests, checking tests on the previously measured specimens and statistical evaluation of results.

b. *Accuracy*
   - It is the closeness of the estimated value to the true mean.
   - Can be checked by the use of reference materials.

Four Components of Quality Assurance

1. Internal quality control (IQC)
2. External quality control (EQC)
3. Standardization
4. Proficiency surveillance

1. Internal Quality Control

- For continuous evaluation of the reliability of the work in laboratory.
- Provides us a way to check precision
- Done by running of internal controls on all the hematology analyzers and daily interpreting and evaluating these results by using routine samples.

2. External Quality Control

- Evaluating the performance of large number of laboratories by an outside agency.
- Organized on a national or regional basis

- *Principle:* Same material is sent from a national or regional center to a large number of laboratories.
- All the laboratories send the results back to the center, where they are analyzed and interpreted.
- When the results are returned from the participants, the median or mean and standard deviation are calculated.
- An individual laboratory can then compare its own performance in the survey with that of other laboratories and also with its own previous performance.

3. Standardization

- Standard values of each test are being followed universally
- These standard values are used for comparing the test results.

4. Proficiency Surveillance

- Includes the critical supervision of all aspects of laboratory tests, before the tests are performed and of reading and reporting of results.
- Also includes maintenance and control of equipment and apparatus.

Control Materials

1. Specially prepared
2. Can be anticoagulated whole blood, preserved pooled red cells, plasma or serum.
3. Should have controls of high, normal and low values.

Analysis of Data

- It is done by standard deviation of the control specimens.
- 95% of the results on the same specimen should be within ±2SD and 99.7% within ± 3SD.
- If measurements are more widely dispersed, it indicates an error in the test.
- Results obtained with the control samples can be plotted on a chart.
- Levey-Jennings chart are most commonly used for interpretation of results.

Maintenance of Hematology Analyzer

Function Check

1. Calibration
   - After major repair
   - New instrument
2. Use of control material.

Maintenance

- Stabilized voltage
- Vibration-free surface
- Dust-free
- Probe damage
- For systematic quality control error.

Cleaning

- Wiping
- Chamber cleaning
- Disinfection: Uusing hypochlorite solution.

Quality Control in Histopathology

Quality control in histopathology can be brought about by coordination between the technical staff and a highly skilled pathologist in histopathology laboratory.

Can be discussed under
- Laboratory quality management system
- Safety control

1. Laboratory Quality Management System
Quality Control
- Provides routine and consistent checks to identify errors.
- Ensures data integrity, correctness and completeness.

What does it ensure?
- Quality control ensures a check on accurate patient identification, fixation, adequate processing, appropriate embedding techniques, microtomy, unacceptable artifacts.
- It also ensures inspection of controls to determine correctness of special stains and immunohistochemical methods.

Whose responsibility is it for this quality control?
It is the responsibility of the pathologist to ensure the check on all these aspects as pathologist is the one who is going to decide, whether the slide is adequate or not for diagnostic interpretation.

How is this quality control plan for histopathology laboratory designed?
Quality control plan should focus on pre-analytical, analytical and post-analytical aspects.

a. *Pre-analytical aspects*
- Include sample collection, transport, and tissue processing and submission of the slide for reporting.
- Standard operating procedure for sample identification, rejection of the sample, and all steps of tissue processing, and staining must be documented and displayed in the laboratory.
- Technical staff should be aware of all these standard operating procedures.
- Stages of fixation, dehydration and clearing must be of sufficient length to ensure completeness.
- Pieces of equipment and instruments in the laboratory should be of standard quality and calibration of these should be done at regular intervals.

b. *Analytical aspects*
- Require the slide interpretation and preparation of report.
- Intradepartmental discussions, expert opinions, external consultations, correlation with history, cytology or frozen reports, all can be done to improve the quality of reporting.

- Protocol preparation for reporting of cancer specimens has proven beneficial for improving the quality of cancer reports.

c. *Post-analytical aspects*
- Preparation and delivery of timely reports.
- Storage of the reported specimen for particular time period followed by safe disposal of the specimen.
- All slides and paraffin blocks should be stored indefinitely, if facilities are available.
- Turnaround time should be maintained by ensuring that reports are being dispatched in shortest time possible.

Turnaround time
a. *For surgical pathology specimens*
- Biopsy—2 days
- Surgical specimen—3 days

Note: Extra-time is allowed for any special procedure done.

b. *For autopsy specimens*
- Provisional report—1 day
- Final report—1 month

2. Safety Control
- All laboratories should enroll in safety programs.
- Safety rules and regulations should be strictly implemented.

Health hazards of chemicals
- Formaldehyde, chloroform, diaxone, chromic acid, basic fuscin, potassium dichromate are all carcinogenic.
- Cyanide and heavy metals can result in acute or chronic poisoning.
- Methanol, chromic acid, osmium tetraoxide are all toxic.
- Xylene and toluene have neurotoxic effects
- Diethyl ether, ethyl alcohol, methyl alcohol and acetone are highly flammable.
- Picric acid is an explosive chemical

Ways through which laboratory workers can get exposed to infectious agents
- Aerosol inhalation
- Contact with non-intact skin
- Contact with mucous membranes

What safety measures should be employed in the laboratories?
- Technical staff should have knowledge of handling, storage and disposal of each solution.
- Only authorized personnel should be allowed in laboratories.
- No eating, drinking, smoking should be allowed.
- Confine long hair and loose clothing
- Avoid mouth pipetting of chemicals or infectious materials.
- Wearing safety glasses and goggles
- Laboratory coats should be completely buttoned
- Work areas should include labels indicating warning signs of fire hazards and various hazardous materials.
- Proper ventilation system should be implemented.
- All laboratory staff should possess the knowledge of first aid.
- Proper spillage methods should be implemented and followed.
- Adequate steps should be taken for proper disposal of toxic and biohazardous substances.

Quality Control Indicators in Surgical Pathology Laboratory

Prospective	• Intradepartmental consultation
	• Interdepartmental consultation
	• Frozen section review
	• Surgical pathology cases random review
	• Autopsy cases random review
Retrospective	• Intradepartmental and interdepartmental conferences
	• Interinstitutional review
	• Specimen adequacy record
	• Lost specimen record
	• Histology slides delivery

External Quality Assurance Programme (EQAP)

In surgical pathology proficiency testing, provider distributes a piece of tissue in a fixative to participant's laboratories.

Following parameters are noted for each participant:

i. Staining quality
ii. Mounting quality
iii. Labeling quality
iv. Description of microscopic findings
v. Final impression
vi. Special staining if performed.

Record Keeping in Laboratory

A. Inspection Records

- Of the laboratory safety audits
- Of the emergency and safety equipment checks
- Hazardous waste inspection reports.

B. Records of Training

- Name of the trainer and date of the class
- Type of training and materials covered in the training.
- Names and signatures of attendees
- Attendance

C. Accident, Injury and Fire Records

- Reports are prepared in case of fire, accidents or injury.

- Also, the cause and nature of the accident and the injuries which it produced should be documented and recorded.
- Records of the steps taken for prevention of the same in future.

D. Exposure Records

Workplace monitoring of toxic substances or harmful physical agents.

E. Other Records

- Samples/specimens, results and issued final report.
- Records of the maintenance and calibration of the equipment.
- Records of all the quality control tests performed to confirm the accuracy of the work.

Role of Medical Laboratory Technology in Healthcare

Medical laboratory technical (MLT) personnel play a role in

a. Assisting physicians in diagnosis and management of the disease.

b. Human and community health

c. Screening of healthy population for various diseases.

d. FNAC techniques, histopathological techniques and hematological techniques.

e. Performing immunohistochemical analysis like ER/PR, which is important for prognostication of breast cancer patients.

f. Achieving and setting goals for "targeted therapy"

g. Performing serum marker studies like PSA, CEA, CA 19-9.

h. Performing various tests for endocrine diseases like HbA1c and TSH.

i. Investigation and surveillance of epidemic diseases.

j. Detection of strains of respiratory viruses or serology for epidemic viral diseases like dengue and chikungunya.

Setting up of a Blood Bank

1. Concerned authority should apply for the place and layout plan approval to the Director of Drugs Control of their respective state.

Guidelines for the space allotment

a. Location should be away from open sewage, drain and unhygienic conditions.

b. Place should be well lighted, ventilated with drains of adequate size to be provided.

c. Minimum area for the blood bank required is 100 sqm for collection, processing, storage and distribution.

d. An additional 50 sqm for preparation of blood components and 10 sqm for apheresis is compulsory.

Rooms in a blood bank should be allotted for

a. Registration and medical examination room for donors

b. Blood collection (air conditioned)

c. Blood component preparation (air conditioned), temperature between 20° and 25°C

d. Laboratory for blood group serology (air conditioned)

e. Serology laboratory for screening of blood transmissible diseases like hepatitis, syphilis, malaria, HIV.

f. Refreshment-cum-rest room (air conditioned)

g. Store-cum-record room

h. Space for toilets (staff and outsiders)

2. After, the site approval is obtained from the Director of Drugs Control (state license authority) blood bank authority should apply for grant of license.

3. Documents to be submitted for grant of license (to operate a blood bank) include:

a. Application form 27C

b. Challan of the fees submitted

c. Declaration form, signed by the head of department

d. Roadmap of the building structure in detail.

e. Attested copies of certificates of qualification, experience, biodata, appointment letter and joining report of medical officer, nurse and technicians employed by the blood bank on regular basis.

f. List of machinery and equipment installed for blood collection and processing.

g. List of component separation units to be started.

h. List of laboratory equipment/apparatus, reagents duly signed by an authorized person/medical officer.

i. NOC from the Pollution Control Board.

Personnel required with their respective qualifications

a. *Medical officer (one)*
   - MD in pathology or transfusion medicine.

- MBBS with diploma in clinical pathology or transfusion medicine with adequate knowledge in blood group serology and medical principles involved in procurement of blood components, or
- MBBS with one year experience in blood banking.

b. *Technician (two)*
   - Degree in MLT with 6 months experience in testing blood/components, or
   - Diploma in MLT with 1 year experience in testing blood and/or components.

c. *Registered nurses (one)*

d. *Technical supervisor (for blood bank components)*
   - Degree in MLT with 6 months experience in component preparation, or
   - Diploma in MLT with 1 year experience in component preparation.

Equipment

1. *General pieces of equipment and instruments (blood collection)*
   a. Donor bed, chair and tables
   b. Bedside table
   c. Sphygmomanometer and stethoscope
   d. Recovery beds for donors
   e. Refrigerators, for storing separately tested and untested blood, maintaining temperature between 2° and 6°C with digital dial thermometer, recording thermograph and alarm device with provision of continuous power supply.
   f. Weighing devices for donor and blood containers.

2. *For hemoglobin demonstration*
   a. Copper sulphate solution (specific gravity:1.053)
   b. Sterile lancet and impregnated alcohol swabs
   c. Capillary tubes
   d. Sahli's hemoglobinometer/calorimetric method

3. *For temperature and pulse determination*
   a. Clinical thermometers
   b. Watch, stopwatch

4. *For blood containers*
   a. Only disposable PVC blood bags shall be used
   b. *Anticoagulants:* Citrate phosphate dextrose adenine (CPDA) solution or citrate phosphate dextrose adenine-1 (CPDA-1)
   Note: 14 ml solution is required for 100 ml of blood.

5. *Emergency equipment/items*
   a. Oxygen cylinder with mask, gauge and pressure regulator.
   b. 5% glucose and normal saline
   c. Disposable sterile syringes and needles of various sizes.
   d. Disposable sterile IV infusion sets
   e. Ampoules of adrenaline, noradrenaline, dexamethasone, metoclopramide injections.
   f. Aspirin

6. *Accessories*
   a. Emesis basin, hemostats, set clamps, sponge forceps, gauze, dressing jars, waste cans.
   b. Cotton balls, adhesive tapes
   c. Denatured spirit, iodine, liquid soap
   d. Autoclave with temperature and pressure indicator.
   e. Incinerator
   f. Stand-by generator

7. *Laboratory equipment*
   a. Refrigerators with continuous power supply (maintaining a temperature of 4–6°)
   b. Microscope
   c. Centrifuge table
   d. Water bath: 37–56°C
   e. Incubator with control
   f. Pipettes
   g. Glass slides
   h. Test tubes
   i. Test tube racks
   j. Insulated containers for transporting blood, between 2° and 10°C temperature, to wards and hospitals.
   k. Filter papers

l. Plain EDTA vials

m. ELISA reader with printer, washer and micropipettes.

8. *Special reagents*

a. Standard blood grouping sera anti-A, anti-B and anti-D with known controls.

b. Reagents for serological test of syphilis

c. Anti-human globulin sera (Coombs' serum)

d. ELISA kits for hepatitis and HIV I and II

9. *Equipment for blood components*

a. Air conditioner

b. Laminar airflow bench

c. Refrigerated centrifuge

d. Plasma expressor

e. Weighing device

f. Artery forceps, scissors

g. Platelet agitator with incubator

h. Deep freezers maintaining a temperature between $-30°$ to $-40°C$.

i. Refrigerated water bath for plasma thawing.

j. Insulated blood bag containers with provisions for storing at appropriate temperature for transport purposes.

Biohazardous Waste Management (Spill Management)

Classification of Spill

- General spillage of infectious material (blood)
- Microorganisms spillage
  - General infectious microbe and spillage of genetically modified micro-organisms
- General chemical spillage
- Mercury spills
- Radioactive spills
- Solvent spillage
- Spillage onto or into equipment
- Dealing with a suspicious substance.

Spill Management

- Handling worker should equip self with gloves, gown and protective eyewear.
- In case of broken glass, glass pieces should be removed by brush and forceps and each piece should be placed in a leak proof sharp container.
- Cover the spill with a cloth towel to soak up as much as blood/fluid as possible.
- Discard the used towel in a biohazard bag
- Proper ventilation of the room should be ensured.

- Pour broad spectrum disinfectant product on the area of the spill and let it soak for 10 minutes.
- Remove the disinfectant from outside towards the center, while scrubbing the area with durable cloth towel.
- Place this towel in a biohazard bag
- Clean thrice the same place with dampened cloth towels, which are discarded in a biohazard bag.
- Allow the area to dry
- Carefully dispose of the personal protective equipment into the plastic bag: Gloves, gown, and glasses.
- Seal the bag and place it into a second bag, then seal it and mark it with a biohazard label.
- Contact local health department for proper disposal.
- One should check his/her body for contamination.
- Thoroughly wash your hands and arms with warm water and disinfectant soap.
- Incident/accident should be properly reported to the organization to prevent future mishaps.

Standard Operating Procedure (SOP)

- Standard operating procedure (SOP) is a document which ensures that the operations are carried out correctly (quality) and with consistency.
- Are written instructions to provide clear guidance on the process, coordination amongst different segments and timely troubleshooting.
- Intended to assist the organization in maintaining quality control and quality assurance process.
- Updated SOPs should be available in writing and in electronic format, and should be readily accessible in the workplace.
- Should be prepared by subject experts
- Should be drafted in a simple, lucid language imparting sufficient details so that it can be easily understood by the personnel performing the procedure.
- They should undergo periodical review and should be kept updated.

Uses

- Imparts consistency in the procedure's outcome.
- Institutional and government regulations are strictly followed.
- To train personnel
- In preventing miscommunications among the staff.

- Address the safety concerns
- Useful in accreditation and auditing processes.

General Format

1. *Title page* should contain the following information:
   - A title clearly identifying the activity or procedure
   - SOP identification (ID) number
   - Date of issue and/or revision
   - Name of the department, division, and/or branch to which SOP applies.
   - Signature with signature dates of those individuals, who prepared and approved the SOP.
2. Table of content
3. Purpose
4. *Responsibilities:*
   - Identify the personnel, who have a primary role in the SOP.
   - Describing these personnel their set of responsibilities.
5. Scope and application
6. *References:* Complete reference should be written.
7. *Definition:* Identify and define frequently used terms.
8. Materials required

9. Procedure
   - Provide the steps required to perform the procedure
10. Results

11. Interpretation
12. Documentation
13. Appendices

Example:

No	Effective date	Pages	Author	Authorized by
SOP/_____	DD/MM/YY	02	xxxxxxxxx	xxxxxxxxx
Versions	Review period	No of copies	Approved by	Date
01	Biennial	02	xxxxxxxxx	DD/MM/YY

Statistical use in a Clinical Laboratory

Validity of the Test

Validity of a test can be measured by two variables:

a. Sensitivity

b. Specificity

Sensitivity: Determines who has the disease. It is the probability that a test is positive when the disease is present.

It is derived by the formula:

$$\text{Sensitivity} = \frac{a}{a + c} = \frac{\text{true positive}}{\text{true positive} + \text{false negative}}$$

	Disease present	Disease absent
Positive for a test	a (True positive)	b (False positive)
Negative for a test	c (False negative)	d (True negative)
Total	**a + c**	**b + d**

Specificity: Identifies those who do not have the disease as really not having the disease. It is a probability that a test is negative when the disease is not present.

It is derived by the formula:

$$\frac{d}{b + d} = \frac{\text{true negative}}{\text{false postive} + \text{true negative}}$$

For example:

	Disease present	Disease absent
Positive for a test	40	5
Negative for a test	20	35
Total	**60**	**40**

Sensitivity = 40/60 = 66.7%

Specificity = 35/40 = 87.5%

Predictive Value of the Test Result

Sensitivity and specificity though determine the positivity and negativity of a test respectively, it does not interpret the positivity and negativity of a result on the individual for that there are 2 more variables:

- Positive predictive value
- Negative predictive value

Positive Predictive Value (PPV)

Determines the probability that the individual has the disease when the test result is positive.

It should be mentioned that a disease is more prevalent in the population will have a more PPV for a given sensitive test.

It is derived by the formula:

$$\frac{a}{a + b} = \frac{\text{true positive}}{\text{true positive} + \text{false positive}}$$

Negative Predictive Value (NPV)

Determines the probability that the individual does not have the disease when the test result is negative.

It is derived by the formula:

$$\frac{d}{c + d} = \frac{\text{true negative}}{\text{false negative} + \text{true negative}}$$

69

Turnaround Time

- It is the time from the receipt of a sample in laboratory till the report is generated.
- In the modern world of evidence-based medicine, service to the patient by hospital or laboratory is assessed by the rapidity of the result delivery as seen by turnaround time (TAT).
- TAT can be divided into following small nine steps:
  a. Ordering
  b. Collection
  c. Identification
  d. Transportation
  e. Separation
  f. Analysis
  g. Reporting
  h. Interpretation
  i. Action
- TAT varies for emergency and routine services and also for different test reports.

Turnaround Time in Histopathology Laboratory

- Smaller specimens are usually fixed by the time, the specimen is received in laboratory.
- Larger specimens require longer fixation before processing.
- According to College of American Pathologists (CAP) guidelines, routine surgical pathology reports should be completed within 2 working days.

- Complicated cases may require additional time for complete processing and/or special studies.
- Large anatomical specimens require more time, due to adequate fixation.
- For bone tissues and biopsies, decalcification of the tissue delays the TAT.
- Additional time is required for lymph node specimens which require immunohistochemical staining.
- Tissues which require deep cuts, recuts, special stain studies or inter- or intra-departmental consultation require more days to report.

Note: Monthly assessment of the departmental surgical pathology laboratory for turnaround time should be done and recorded by the concerned pathologist, any deficits, if found, should be corrected upon for improving of turnaround time for future reports.

Steps to Reduce Turnaround Time in a Laboratory

Pre-analytical phase
1. Adoption of ideal phlebotomy practices.
2. Use of computer generated requisition slips.
3. Accessioning of the samples can be done by bar code readers.
4. Specimen should be transported rapidly from collection centers to laboratory area,

which can be done by the help of pneumatic system.

Analytical phase

5. Use of fully automated machines with higher throughput.
6. Adoption of efficient quality control procedures and updated standard operating protocols.
7. Training of technical staff to handle urgent samples with priority.

Post-analytical phase

8. Adoption of laboratory information system (LIS) for the validation of reports.
9. Dispatch the reports through the information system software, which should be made easily accessible to the treating physicians in wards, emergency rooms and operation theaters.
10. Interaction with the customers and paying attention to their feedbacks to improve TAT.

Methods of Disposal of Pathological Waste

Pathological Waste

- Includes biopsy materials, human tissues, anatomical parts from surgery and other procedures.
- Also includes carcasses and bedding from the animals exposed to pathogens in research.
- Pathological waste must be incinerated.

Hospital waste categories and disposal of human waste are given below.

WHO Medical Waste Categories

A. *Infectious (Materials Containing Pathogens if Exposed can Cause Disease)*

- Human anatomical waste: Waste from surgery and autopsies on the patients with infectious diseases.
- Sharps: Disposable needles, syringes, saws, blades, broken glasses, nails or any other item that could cause a cut.
- Pathological: Tissues, organs, body parts, human flesh, fetuses, blood and body fluids.

Category	Waste category	Treatment and disposal
I	Human anatomical waste	Incineration/deep burial
II	Animal waste	Incineration/deep burial
III	Microbiology and biotechnology waste	Incineration/deep burial
IV	Sharps	Incineration/disinfection/chemical treatment/mutilation
V	Medicine and cytotoxic drugs	Incineration/destruction and disposal in secured landfill
VI	Solid waste (blood and body fluids)	Autoclave/chemical treatment/burial
VII	Solid waste (disposable items)	Autoclave/chemical treatment/burial
VIII	Liquid waste (blood and body fluids)	Disinfection by chemicals/discharge into drains
IX	Incineration ash	Disposal in municipal landfill
X	Chemical waste	Chemical treatment/secure landfill

B. *Non-infectious (Hazardous)*

- *Pharmaceuticals:* Drugs and chemicals that are returned from wards, spilled, outdated, contaminated, or are no longer required.
- *Radioactive:* Solids, liquids and gaseous waste contaminated with radioactive substances used in diagnosis and treatment of diseases like toxic goiter.

C. *Non-infectious (Non-hazardous)*

Domestic waste from the offices, kitchens, rooms, including bed-linen, utensils, paper, etc.

Segregation of the Waste by Color Coding System

Three categories:

1. Infectious waste—red bags
2. Domestic waste—green bags
3. Sharps—needle cutters/punctureproof containers.

Transportation

a. *Containers:* Punctureproof, leakproof
b. *Bags:* Sturdy, properly tied
c. *Transport trolleys:* Designated and timely
d. *Staff protection:* Provided with protective clothing and other items.

Note

- Never put hands in a bag
- Infectious material in red bags will go for incineration.
- Sharps can either go to incinerator or following autoclaving/chemical disinfection can be mutilated.

Note: For details, go through the topic of biomedical waste management of this book.

Section
V

Clinical Pathology

Chapters

Fluids

CEREBROSPINAL FLUID (CSF)

Collection

CSF should be collected and received in laboratory in sterile tubes as follows:

Tube 1: For glucose and protein estimation and serological examination.

Tube 2: For microbiological examination (Gram's staining, bacterial culture and sensitivity)

Tube 3: Hematology (total cell count and differential count)

Tube 4: Cytology and special studies

Note: CSF should be examined within 1 hour of collection and CSF cell counts are done within 30–60 minutes.

A. How to Proceed for Cell Count in a Hematology Laboratory?

Cell count should be done immediately after receiving the sample as the cells starts degenerating rapidly.

1. *Total Leukocyte Count*

Methods

- CSF should be properly mixed
- If CSF sample appears clear grossly, no diluent is used.
- However, if CSF appears turbid, 1:20 dilution is made using 0.05 ml of CSF and 0.95 ml of Türk solution (Türk fluid is composed of glacial acetic acid 4 ml, methylene blue solution 10 drops, and distilled water to make 200 ml).
- Fluid is charged on a Neubauer counting chamber, which is covered with the coverslip.
- After charging the chamber, fluid is allowed to stand for 2 minutes for cells to settle.
- *Note:* For counting cells in CSF, Fuchs-Rosenthal counting chamber is preferred because its depth is twice that of improved Neubauer chamber.
- *Normal cell count:* (a) Adult = 0 to 5/mm^3, (b) newborn = 0 to 30 /mm^3, (c) child = 0 to 15/ mm^3.

2. *Differential Leukocyte Count*

- CSF cells should be studied on a slide following a cytospin preparation and centrifugation should not be done as it results in cell disintegration.
- In normal adults, differential count shows 70% lymphocytes and 30% monocytes.

Interpretation (Table 71.1)

- Increased neutrophils are seen in bacterial meningitis.
- Increased lymphocytes are seen in tubercular and viral meningitis.

Table 71.1: CSF findings in different types of meningitis

Condition	Leukocytes	Proteins (mg/dl)	Glucose (mg/dl)
1. Normal	<5 μl (mostly lymphocytes)	15–45	45–80
2. Acute pyogenic meningitis	Increased	Increased	Decreased
3. Tuberculous meningitis	Increased	Increased	Decreased
4. Viral meningitis	Increased	Increased	Normal

B. Chemical Examination

1. *Estimation of proteins in CSF*
   - Turbidimetric method: Trichloroacetic acid when added to the CSF results in precipitation of proteins with resultant turbid solution.
   - Normal levels in adults: 15–45 mg/dl
2. *Estimation of glucose in CSF:*
   - CSF glucose is measured by glucose oxidase method.
   - Normal range: 45–80 mg/dl.

C. Microbiological Examination

1. *Direct wet mount of CSF for cryptococcosis:* One drop of CSF deposit (obtained after centrifugation) is placed on a glass slide, covered with a cover glass and examined under the microscope.
2. *Ziehl-Neelsen smear:* If tuberculosis meningitis is suspected.
3. Culture for bacteria and *Mycobacterium tuberculosis.*
4. PCR for *Mycobacterium tuberculosis* and viruses.

PLEURAL FLUID

- Pleural cavity is a space between the chest wall and the lungs, on both sides.
- It contains a small amount of fluid (<10 ml) in normal individuals.
- Normal pleural fluid is clear and straw or pale yellow in color.
- *Pleural effusion:* Accumulation of excess fluid in pleural cavity.

Fluid Collection

- Aspiration of fluid from the pleural space is called thoracocentesis.

- *For diagnostic studies:* Fluid should be collected in heparinized tubes to prevent clotting.
- *For cell counts:* Sample is collected in EDTA anticoagulant.
- *For microbiological studies:* Sterile sample tubes should be used.

Cell Counts in Pleural Fluid Samples

- Take the sample in test tube and dilute it with Türk's fluid, the sample and Türk's fluid are taken in equal proportions.
- Following dilution, Neubauer's chamber is charged for cell count.
- For cytological examination, pleural fluid is centrifuged, smears are prepared from the sediment and are stained with Leishman stain.

Other Tests

- Gram's stain
- Ziehl-Neelsen stain
- Culture

PERITONEAL FLUID/ASCITIC FLUID

- Peritoneal cavity is a space in the abdominal cavity lined by mesothelial cells.
- This cavity normally contains 30–50 ml of serous fluid.
- Pathological accumulation of fluid in the cavity is called ascites and the accumulated fluid is called ascitic fluid.

Examination of the Ascitic Fluid

Tests are commonly performed on ascitic fluid.

1. White Cell Count

- Elevated neutrophil count suggests bacterial infection.

- Elevated lymphocyte count suggests peritoneal tuberculosis or malignancy.

2. Chemical Examination

a. *Albumin*

- Serum to ascites albumin gradient is calculated by subtracting ascites albumin from serum albumin (gm/dl).
- Classified into high albumin gradient (>1.1) ascites and low albumin gradient (<1.1) ascites.

b. Lactate dehydrogenase levels

c. Amylase levels

d. Bilirubin

3. Microbiological Examination

- Gram-positive organisms can be isolated in blood culture bottles.
- Ziehl-Neelsen stain is used for diagnosing *Mycobacterium tuberculosis*.

4. Cytological Examination

For diagnosing malignant cells in ascitic fluid.

Semen Analysis

Semen is a fluid, which contains sperms that fertilize the female ova.

Semen volume is contributed by testes, epididymis, vas deferens, seminal vesicles, prostate and Cowper glands.

Indications for Semen Analysis

- Investigation for infertility
- For checking the effectiveness of vasectomy by confirming the absence of sperms.
- For paternity issues
- For medicolegal cases, e.g. in cases of rape
- For selection of donors in reproductive technology.
- For selection of assisted reproductive techniques.

Semen Collection

- Semen specimen is collected after 3 days of abstinence.
- Longer period of abstinence reduces the sperm motility and shorter duration of abstinence reduces sperm count.
- Sample is obtained by masturbation in clean, dry, sterile, and wide-mouthed plastic container.
- Sample should be brought to laboratory within 1 hour of collection.
- If transportation is necessary, specimen should be kept close to body temperature.
- Condom collection is not advisable as condom contains spermicidal agents.

Semen analysis should include:

a. *Physical examination:* Liquefaction time of semen, viscosity, volume of the semen, pH of the semen and its color.
b. Microscopic examination for sperm count, sperm motility, sperm morphology and sperm vitality (live sperms) and proportion of WBCs.
c. *Biochemical analysis:* Fructose, zinc, acid phosphatase.
d. *Immunological analyses:* Anti-sperm antibodies.
e. *Bacteriological analysis:* Detection of infection.

A. Physical Examination (Salient Features)

- Normal semen is viscous and opaque gray white.
- Normal semen is thick and liquefies within 30 minutes by the action of prostatic enzymes.
- Viscosity is assessed by filling a pipette with semen and allowing it to flow in a container. Normal semen will fall drop by drop and if the droplets form threads more than 2 cm long, it indicates viscosity is increased.
- Volume of the semen collected should be 2 ml.
- Normal pH of semen is 7.2 to 8 after an hour of ejaculation.

B. Microscopic Examination

1. Sperm Motility

- *Principle:* All motile and non-motile sperms are counted in wet preparation smear.
- *Method:* Drop of semen is placed on a glass slide, covered with a coverslip, and 200 sperms are counted.

2. Sperm Vitality

- For counting live sperms and dead sperms with eosin and nigrosin stain.
- Principle: A cell with intact cell membrane will not take up eosin Y and will not be stained, while a dead sperm with damaged cell membrane, will take up the dye and is stained pink red.

Methods

- Mix one drop of semen with one drop of eosin–nigrosin solution and incubate for 30 seconds.
- Smear is made from drop placed on a glass slide.
- Smear is air-dried and examined under oil-immersion objective. White sperms are classified as live or viable and red sperms are classified as dead or non-viable.

3. Sperm Count

Principle: Sperm count is done after liquefaction in a counting chamber following dilution and number of spermatozoa are reported in millions/millimeter.

Methods

- Semen is diluted 1:20 with sodium bicarbonate-formalin diluting fluid (take 1 ml of semen in a graduated tube and fill with diluting fluid to 20 ml mark and mix them well).
- Neubauer's chamber is charged with above prepared diluted semen sample with the help of Pasteur's pipette.
- Following which the chamber is kept in a humid box for the sperms to settle down.
- Count is done on the large four corner squares.
- >20 million/ml is normal sperm count.

4. Sperm Morphology

- A smear is prepared by spreading a drop of seminal fluid on a glass slide, stained and percentages of normal and abnormal forms of spermatozoa are counted.
- Stains employed can be Papanicolaou stain, eosin stain and nigrosin stain, hematoxylin and eosin and toluidine blue stain.
- At least 200 spermatozoa should be counted under oil immersion.
- Normally, >30% of sperms should show normal morphology.

5. Round Cells

- On microscopic examination, they may be white blood cells or immature sperm cells.
- Papanicolaou stain is used to differentiate between them.

C. Biochemical Analysis of Semen

Test for fructose

- Resorcinol method is used detection of fructose.
- 5 ml of resorcinol reagent is added to 0.5 ml of seminal fluid. Mixture is heated and brought to boil. If fructose is present, a red color precipitate is formed within 30 seconds.

Sputum Examination

Sputum examination refers to the examination of the material coughed out from the lungs, bronchi, trachea, and larynx.

Role of Sputum Examination

- Identification of the causative organism in lower respiratory tract infection, e.g. pneumonia, suspected tuberculosis, fungal infection, *Pneumocystis carinii* pneumonia in HIV individuals, bronchiectasis.
- Cytological examination for malignant cells.

Collection of Sputum

- Sputum sample should be collected in morning, soon after awakening (as secretions accumulate overnight).
- Sputum is collected in a clean, dry, wide-mouthed container, with a tight cap and a capacity of 25 ml.
- It is advisable for the patient to take deep breath, and cough deeply before spitting in the container. 2–5 ml of sputum is collected.
- For microbiological studies, sample should be sent to the laboratory immediately.
- For distant transportation, sputum should be collected in 25 ml of the following solution:
  - N-acetylpyridinium chloride 5 gm
  - Sodium chloride 10 gm
  - Distilled water up to 1000 ml

1. Microbiological Examination

A. Gram Staining

Pathogenic organisms found in sputum include:

a. *Gram-positive: Streptococcus pneumoniae, Streptococcus pyogenes, Staphylococcus aureus.*
b. *Gram-negative: Haemophilus influenzae, Klebsiella pneumoniae, Pseudomonas aeruginosa, Yersinia pestis, Moraxella catarrhalis.*

Sample processing

- For bacteriological examination, sputum sample should be processed within 1 hour of collection.
- A thin smear is made on a glass slide from the sputum with a clean stick, which is air-dried, fixed and stained with Gram's stain.

B. Bacteriological Culture

- Portion of the purulent sputum is inoculated on the culture medium for identification of organisms.
- Sputum is washed with normal saline to wash away saliva.
- Washed sputum is inoculated on (a) blood agar plate, (b) chocolate agar plate.
- The blood agar plate and chocolate agar plate are incubated.
- These incubated plates are inspected for growth after 18 hours, if growth is not satisfactory, incubation for further 24 hours is indicated.

2. Examination of Sputum for Mycobacterium Tuberculosis

Tests to detect tuberculosis on sputum

a. Examination of sputum smears by Ziehl-Neelsen technique and fluorescence microscopy.
b. Culture on conventional medium
c. Automated culture systems
d. Molecular methods

a. Examination of Sputum Smears

- For detection of *Mycobacterium tuberculosis*, at least three sputum samples are collected and examined, including one early morning specimen.
- A thin smear is prepared on a clean glass slide from yellowish portion of the sputum.
- Smear is stained with Ziehl-Neelsen (ZN) stain and examined under light microscopy, or
- Auramine-rhodamine or auramine O, fluorochrome dyes can be used to highlight bacteria in a smear, if fluorescent microscope is available.
- With ZN stain, Mycobacterium appears as bright red straight or slightly curved beaded rods (2–4 micron in length and 0.2–0.5 micron in width) against a blue background.
- Mycobacteria are both acid and alcohol-fast bacilli and are termed acid-fast bacilli.

Note: ZN stain sputum smear is positive, if at least 5000–10000 tubercle bacilli/ml are present in sputum.

b. Culture

- More sensitive than sputum smear examination
- Can detect 10–100 microorganisms per ml of sputum sample.
- It is an expensive test and requires 6 weeks for its result.

Culture Medium used for Isolation of Tuberculosis

a. *Solid medium:* Egg based (Lowenstein-Jensen medium) or agar based (Middlebrook 7H10)
b. *Liquid medium:* Middlebrook 7H9, Middlebrook 7H12.

Most commonly used solid medium for culture is Lowenstein-Jensen medium and Mycobacterium requires 6 weeks for its growth.

Important Points to Remember

- Freshly collected sputum sample should be sent immediately to the laboratory without addition of any fixative.
- In cases of delay, Saccomano's fixative is used for fixation, which comprises mixture of 50% ethyl alcohol and 2% carbowax.

Stool Examination

Following are the indications for stool examination:

a. *Detection of parasites:* For detection of adult worms, tapeworms, larva, ova
b. *Evaluation of diarrhea*
   - Chronic diarrhea refers to the passage of 3 or more loose or liquid stools per day for more than 4 weeks.
   - Acute diarrhea is defined as passage of 3 or more loose or liquid stools per day for less than 4 weeks.
c. *Evaluation of dysentery:* For identification of the causative organism and differentiating amebic from bacillary dysentery.
d. *Bacteriological examination:* Infection by bacteria such as Salmonella, Shigella, Vibrio, Yersinia, or *Clostridium difficile* can be identified by stool culture.
e. *Chemical examination:* Chemical tests can be applied on feces to detect blood, fat and urobilinogen.
f. *For diagnosing rotavirus:* Rotavirus can be identified by examination of stool by immunofluorescence, or ELISA.

Microscopic Examination

A. Collection of Specimen for Parasites

- 20–40 gm of formed stool or 5–6 tablespoons of watery stool should be collected and is transported immediately to the laboratory.
- In cases of delay in examination of feces, sample must be refrigerated.
- A fixative containing 10% formalin may be used, if the specimen is to be transported to a distant laboratory.
- One negative report for ova and parasites does not exclude the possibility of the infection.
- Three separate samples, collected at 3-day intervals, are recommended to detect all parasite infections.

Preparation of slides
- After receipt in laboratory, saline and iodine wet mounts of the sample are prepared.
- A drop of normal saline is placed near one end of the glass slide and a drop of Lugol's iodine solution is placed near the other end.
- A small amount of feces is mixed with a drop of each saline and iodine using a wire-loop and a coverslip is placed over each preparation, separately.

Saline wet mount is used for demonstration of:
- Eggs and larva of helminths
- Trophozoites and cysts of protozoa
- Can detect RBCs and WBCs
- Iodine stains glycogen and nuclei of the cysts.

Iodine wet mount is used for identification of protozoal cysts.

B. *Test for Occult Blood in Stools*

- Occult blood means presence of blood in feces, which is not obvious grossly.
- Screening procedure for detection of colorectal carcinoma.
    1. *Tests for detection of occult blood in feces:* Tests based on peroxidase like activity of hemoglobin: Benzidine, orthotoluidine method.
    2. *Immunochemical tests:* Test contains mixing of the sample with latex particles coated with anti-human hemoglobin antibody. Presence of agglutination indicates positive results.
    3. *Radioisotope test using chromium 51*

C. *Test for Presence of Fat in Feces*

Microscopic stool examination after staining for fat: Stool sample is stained with a fat stain (oil red O, Sudan III or Sudan IV) and is observed under the microscope for fat globules.

D. *Test for Urobilinogen in Feces*

- Fecal urobilinogen is determined by Ehrlich's aldehyde test.
- Normal amount of urobilinogen excreted in feces is 50–300 mg/day.

E. *Test for Reducing Sugars*

Benedict's test or Clinitest tablet test is used to detect sugars in freshly collected stool sample.

Collection and Processing of Urine

A. Collection of Urine Sample

- First voided morning, midstream specimen, is most concentrated and has acidic pH.
- This specimen is used for routine and microscopic examination.

24-hour Urine Specimen Collection

- Used for quantitative estimation of proteins and hormones.
- After discarding the first voided urine sample, urine should be collected throughout the day and also the next day morning first urine sample is collected.
- Urine should be preserved at 4–6°C and is immediately transported to the laboratory.

What are the Various Collection Methods?

- *Midstream specimen collection of urine:* First half of the stream acts to flush out the contaminating cells and microbes, subsequent stream is collected.
- *Catheter specimen:* Used for bedridden and ill patients, or patients with urinary tract obstruction.
- *Infants:* Suprapubic aspiration, by passing a needle into the bladder, just above the symphysis pubis.

B. Preservation of Urine Sample

Chemical preservatives added to 24-hour urine samples: Hydrochloric acid, toluene, boric acid, thymol, formalin.

Note: Urine sample should be tested in a laboratory within 2 hours of collection for correct results.

Urine Examination in Detail

A. *Gross or Physical Examination*

1. *Appearance: Color:* Yellow—urochrome, pale—excessive fluid intake, red—hematuria (RBCs in urine), hemoglobinuria (hemoglobin in urine), yellow brown—bile pigments, orange red—urobilin
2. *Volume:* Normal volume—600–2000 ml/day, polyuria—>2000 ml/day, oliguria—<500 ml/day.
3. *Specific gravity*
   - Normal adults: 1.016–1.022/24 hours
   - Methods to measure specific gravity—reagent strip method, urinometer, falling drop method.
   a. *Reagent strip method*
      - Reagent strip comprises polyelectrolyte, indicator substance and buffer.
      - The indicator substance of the strip than changes color because of the pH change of polyelectrolytes in relation to the ionic concentration of the urine.
   b. *Urinometer*
      - Measures the specific gravity at room temperature.
      - Urinometer vessel is filled with 15 ml of urine and the urinometer is inserted

with a spinning rotation, so that it should not touch the sides or the bottom of the cylinder and specific gravity reading is measured at the lower meniscus.

Note: Falling drop method and refractometer requires only few drops of urine for determining the specific gravity of the sample.

4. *Urine pH:* In normal individuals, urine pH varies from 4.6 to 8.

Methods

- Reagent strip method: Using a reagent strip
- Litmus paper test: Alkaline urine turns red litmus paper to blue and acidic urine turns blue litmus paper to red.

B. Chemical Examination

1. *Proteins*

150 mg of protein is excreted daily in urine. Albumin makes one-third of its composition

Methods to detect proteins

a. *Reagent strip method:* Semi-quantitative test, can detect only albumin.
b. *Sulfosalicyclic acid test*
   - Semi-quantitative test
   - Principle: Cold precipitation of urine
   - Take 2.5 ml of urine in a test tube and add similar amount of sulfosalicylic acid. Invert to mix. Wait for 5 minutes. Using ordinary room light the turbidity is assessed and graded.
   - Test results can vary from: Negative (no turbidity), trace (perceptible turbidity), 1+ (distinct turbidity), 2+ (turbidity with granulation), 3+ (turbidity with flocculation), 4+ (clumps of protein).
c. *Heat and acetic acid test*
   - Principle: Heat-induced coagulation of proteins
   - Take urine in a test tube, and fill three-fourths of it, heat upper one-third of the urine sample. The lower part is taken as control for checking the turbidity in the

upper heated part. Do not boil it, as it results in mixing of the upper and lower parts of the urine.

- Interpretation: Development of turbidity may be due to coagulation of proteins or due to phosphates. Add 5 drops of 10% glacial acetic acid, it will dissolve the phosphates and if the turbidity persists in the urine sample, it is because of proteins.

2. *Glucose in urine*

- In hyperglycemia, glycosuria occurs when the blood glucose is 180–200 mg/dl.
- In diabetic patients, glucose measurement in urine is easy and inexpensive.

Methods to detect glucose in urine

a. *Reagent strip test:* Components include glucose oxidase, peroxidase and chromogen (*o*-toluidine and potassium iodide)
   - Glucose + O_2 (glucose oxidase) → gluconic acid and H_2O_2
   - H_2O_2 + chromogen (peroxidase) → oxidized chromogen + H_2O
   - *Interpretation:* If color change in the reagent strip is noted, the urine sample contains glucose.
b. *Copper reduction test*
   - Detects any reducing substance in urine, including reducing sugars like lactose, fructose, galactose, and maltose.

Benedict's test

Principle: Copper sulfate in Benedict's reagent reacts with reducing substances in urine which convert cupric sulphate (Cu^{2+}) to cuprous oxide (Cu^{3+}) in hot alkaline medium.

Procedure

- Take 5 ml of Benedict's reagent in a test tube and boil to exclude reducing substances. Add 8 drops (0.5 ml) of urine. Boil the mixture for 5 minutes and cool.
- If the color changes from blue to green, it indicates presence of sugar in urine.

- Depending on the amount of sugar present, color change varies from green precipitate followed by yellow precipitate, orange precipitate and brick red precipitate in increasing order of severity.

3. *Ketones in urine*
- Includes acetoacetic acid (normal levels: <2 mg/dl), acetone (normal levels: 17–42 mg/dl) and beta-hydroxybutyric acid.
- Seen in diabetes patients, in whom, up to 50 mg/dl of acetoacetic acid can be seen in urine, a condition called diabetic ketonuria.

Methods
a. *Reagent strip method*
b. *Rothera's test*
  - *Principle:* Acetoacetic acid and acetone react with sodium nitroprusside in presence of alkali to form purple color compound.
  - Take 4 ml of urine in a test tube, and add a few crystals of sodium nitroprusside and saturate the urine with ammonium sulfate by mixing vigorously. Overlay with a few drops of liquor ammonia along the wall of the tube.
  - *Result:* Purple ring indicates the presence of acetoacetic acid or acetone.
c. *Gerhardt's test/ferric chloride test*
  - In 8 ml of urine, add 10% of ferric chloride solution drop by drop, till a precipitate of ferric phosphate forms.
  - Add more ferric chloride solution till the ferric phosphate precipitate disappears.
  - Filter it and add 1–2 more drops of ferric chloride to the filtrate.
  - *Interpretation:* A red color of the filtrate indicates positive test.
  - Detects only acetoacetic acid

4. *Bilirubin in urine:* Bilirubin is usually absent in urine, and its presence indicates obstructive jaundice.
   a. *Dipstick method:* Based on diazo reaction
   b. *Fouchet's test*

- Fouchet's reagent contains trichloroacetic acid and ferric chloride.
- In an acidic medium, ferric chloride oxidizes bilirubin to produce a dark green-colored biliverdin.

Procedure
- In 10 ml of urine, add 3 ml of barium chloride solution.
- Mix the two and filter
- On filter paper, bilirubin and barium salt remains.
- On the filter paper, add a few drops of Fouchet's reagent.
- *Interpretation:* Green/blue color indicates bilirubinuria.

5. *Bile salts:* These are glycine and taurine salts of cholic acid and chenodeoxycholic acid.

Hay's sulfur test
Principle: Bile salts have property of lowering surface tension of urine.

Procedure: 10 ml of urine in wide bore conical flask tube (2 cm diameter or more), sprinkle sulfur powder over its surface and wait for 5 minutes.

Result: Sulfur powder sinks down to bottom of the test tube in presence of bile salts in urine.

6. *Hemoglobin in urine*
a. *Reagent strip test*

Principle: Hemoglobin lysis releases heme which has peroxidase like activity which liberates oxygen from peroxide in reagent strip. Oxygen combines with the chromogen and forms colored compound.
1. Peroxide (H_2O_2) $\xrightarrow{\text{Peroxidase}}$ $H_2O + O$
2. O + chromogen (orthotoluidine/tetramethylbenzene) → oxidized chromogen (colored compound)

b. *Benzidine test*
Principle: Hemoglobin releases heme which has peroxidase like activity which causes oxidation of benzidine.

Procedure

- Dissolve small amount of benzidine in mixture of 2 ml of glacial acetic acid + 2 ml of hydrogen peroxide.
- Now from the solution above, take 2 ml of solution into another test tube and add 2 ml of previously boiled and cooled urine and mix.
- *Interpretation:* Appearance of blue color indicates blood.

C. Microscopic Examination

Procedure

- A well-mixed sample of urine is centrifuged in a centrifuge tube for 5 minutes at 1500 rpm and supernatant is poured off.
- From the bottom of the tube, take the sediment in form of a drop, which is placed on a glass slide and covered with a cover-slip.
- The slide is examined immediately under the microscope.

Cytological analysis of urine specimen is done for the assessment of:

a. Red blood cells

b. White blood cells

c. Renal tubular epithelial cells

d. Squamous epithelial cells

e. Transitional epithelial cells

f. *Casts*
  - Are originated from the kidney
  - Have parallel sides and blunt ends
  - Can appear as cylinders
  - *Classification:* Matrix casts (hyaline, waxy), cellular casts (RBC, WBC, tubular epithelial cell casts and mixed casts), inclusion casts.

g. *Crystals*
  - Crystals found in normal acidic urine: Amorphous urates (calcium, magnesium, sodium, potassium), crystalline urates (sodium, potassium, ammonium), crystalline uric acid, calcium oxalates.
  - Crystals found in normal alkaline urine: Amorphous phosphates (calcium, magnesium), crystalline phosphates (triple phosphates), calcium carbonate, ammonium biurate.
  - Crystals found in abnormal urine: Cystine, tyrosine.

Section VI

Transfusion Medicine

Blood Group Systems

- In transfusion medicine, most common blood group systems are ABO and Rh.
- This is because A, B and RhD antigens are immunogenic (i.e. they can elicit a strong antibody response on stimulation).

ABO System

- Four main types of blood groups: A, B, AB, O
- These blood groups are determined on the basis of presence or absence of A and/ or B antigens on RBCs.
- If the antigen is absent in an individual, corresponding antibody is always present in plasma.
- O blood group is commonest, and AB group is least common.

ABO Blood Groups

Blood group	Antigen on RBC	Antibody in plasma
A	A	Anti-B
B	B	Anti-A
AB	AB	Nil
O	Nil	Anti-A or anti-B

Blood Group A

- Antigens present on the RBCs are A and H (common antigen, from which all other antigens are derived from the gene)
- Plasma contains anti-B antibodies.

Blood Group B

- Antigens present on RBCs are B and H
- Plasma contains anti-A antibodies.

Blood Group AB

- Antigens present on RBCs are A, B, and H
- Plasma does not show anti-A or anti-B antibodies.

Blood Group O

- Antigen present on RBCs is H
- Plasma shows anti-A, anti-B and anti-AB antibodies.

Bombay Blood Group

- H gene, which gives rise to H antigen is responsible for formation of A antigen and B antigen on RBCs.
- H antigen + N-acetylgalactosamine = A antigen
- H antigen + galactose = B antigen
- In absence of H antigen in an individual, A and B are not expressed on their RBCs.
- These individuals are said to have Bombay blood group and these people lack H, A and B antigens on their RBCs.

Universal Blood Donor and Recipient

- RBCs of blood group O donors are devoid of A and B antigens and cannot be agglutinated by anti-A and anti-B antibodies, hence individuals with blood group O are considered as universal donors.

- Blood group AB individuals are considered as universal recipients.

The Rh System

- Antigen is called Rh factor, derived from rhesus monkey red cells.
- Discovered by Stetson and Levine
- Antibody against this antigen is called anti-D antibody.

Antigens of Rh System

- D antigen is most immunogenic
- Presence of D antigen, makes an individual Rh positive, while its absence makes an individual Rh negative.
- In India, 95% people express D antigen on their RBCs (Rh positive), while 5% are Rh D negative.

- Rh antigens are expressed only on RBCs and not on any other tissues and are neither secreted in body fluids (unlike ABO antigens).

Rh Antibodies

- Are of IgG class and can induce hemolytic disease of newborn (HDN).
- Thus, in reproductive age group, Rh –ve women, should always be transfused only with Rh negative blood.
- If we transfuse, Rh +ve blood to Rh –ve women, this may result in formation of anti-D antibodies in the female.
- During pregnancy, these IgG anti-D can cross the placenta and induce hemolytic disease of newborn (HDN).
- This HDN can be prevented with immunization of Rh immune globulin to all Rh –ve women during mid-pregnancy and within 72 hours of delivery.

Blood Grouping

ABO GROUPING

A. Forward Grouping (Cell Grouping)

RBCs are tested for the presence of A and B antigens using known specific anti-A and anti-B sera.

B. Reverse Grouping (Serum Grouping)

Serum is tested for the presence of anti-A and anti-B antibodies by group A and group B reagent RBCs.

Three methods for blood grouping: Tube, slide and micro-plate method.

1. *Slide test*
- Red cells of the test sample are reacted with reagent anti-sera (anti-A and anti-B).
- Agglutination of red cells indicates presence of corresponding antigen on RBCs.

Methods

- Clean slide is divided into two portions, which are labeled as anti-A and anti-B.
- On these labeled portions, one drop of anti-A serum and anti-B serum are placed.
- Now, one drop of blood sample to be tested is added to each drop of antiserum.
- Mix antiserum and blood by using a stick
- After thorough tilting the slides and mixing, look for agglutination after 2 minutes.

Results

Positive: Clumps of RBCs (agglutination) seen.
Negative: RBCs clumping is not visualized.

Interpretation

Anti-A	Anti-B	Blood group
+	−	A
−	+	B
+	+	AB
−	−	O

2. *Tube method*
3. *Micro-plate method*

RH D GROUPING

- D antigen should always be detected after ABO antigen detection.
- Presence of D antigen makes an individual as Rh positive and absence of D antigen makes an individual as Rh negative.
- If Rh +ve blood is given to Rh −ve individuals, these individuals will develop anti-Rh D antibodies.
- In pregnant women, these anti-D antibodies can cross the placenta during pregnancy and destroy fetal RBCs and result in hemolytic disease of newborn (HDN).
- Patients red cells are mixed with anti-D reagent.
- Principle of Rh typing is similar to ABO grouping and it is performed at the same time as ABO grouping.

Blood Banking

- Blood donation can be voluntary, replacement or professional.
- A blood donor questionnaire and consent form needs to be filled by the blood donor before donation.

Criteria for Selection of Blood Donors

1. *Age group:* 18–60 years
2. *Donation interval:* Interval between two successive donations should be at least 3 months.
3. *Volume of donation:* Donor weighing 45 kg or more can give 350 ml of blood.
4. *Infectious diseases*
   - HIV individuals should be permanently deferred for donation of blood.
   - Viral hepatitis patients (if there is a history defer the patient for 1 year and HBsAg or anti-HCV positive subjects should be permanently deferred)
   - Malaria infection individuals should be deferred till 3 months.
5. *Illness:* Diabetes mellitus, hypertension, heart disease, renal disease, liver disease, lung disease, cancer, epilepsy, bleeding disorder, allergic disorder are contra-indications for blood donation.
6. *Medications:* Patients on aspirin, anti-cancer drugs are deferred.
7. *Dental treatment:* After dental treatment, blood donation should be carried out only after 72 hours.
8. *Skin piercing:* From any cause, should result in deferral for 12 months.
9. *Blood transfusion:* Individual who has received blood transfusion within last 12 months should be deferred.
10. *Immunization*
    - Hepatitis B immunoglobulin vaccine defers for 1 year
    - Live virus vaccines for measles, mumps, yellow fever, oral polio defer for 2 weeks.
11. *Physical examination*
    - Donor should be in good health
    - Should weigh minimum of 45 kg
    - *Systolic BP:* 100–180 mm Hg and *diastolic BP:* 50–100 mm Hg
    - *Pulse* rate should be 60–100/min and regular
    - *Temperature:* Normal
    - Skin of donor at site of venepuncture should be free of needle prick scars.
12. *Hemoglobin:* Should be more than or equal to 12.5 gm%.

COLLECTION OF DONOR BLOOD

Equipment and Materials

Blood Bags

- Blood is collected in a sterile, disposable plastic bag (single, double, or triple).
- Double and triple bags are used when component separation is required.

- Bags contain 49 ml of citrate phosphate dextrose adenine (CPDA) solution.
- In CPDA-1 solution, blood can be stored at 2–6° C for 35 days.
- CPDA-1 solution inhibits the clotting of blood.

Microorganisms Transmissible by Transfusion

Viruses

- Hepatitis B, C viruses
- HIV 1 and 2
- Parvovirus B19
- Cytomegalovirus

Bacteria

Treponema pallidum

Parasite

Malarial parasite, *Trypanosoma cruzi*, *Toxoplasma gondii*, *Leishmania donovani*.

Mandatory Infectious Disease Testing to be Done in Blood Transfusion Practice in India

1. Syphilis—VDRL test
2. Hepatitis B—HBsAg (hepatitis B surface antigen)
3. Human immunodeficiency virus (HIV) infection—anti-HIV 1 and anti-HIV 2 antibodies.
4. Hepatitis C—anti-HCV antibodies
5. Malaria—peripheral smear.

79

Crossmatching

- Also known as compatibility testing
- Important to perform, before a blood transfusion is given.
- *Aim:* To detect ABO incompatibility between donor and recipient.

Two Types

Major and minor crossmatching:
- *Major crossmatch:* Mixing the patient's plasma with donor's RBCs.
- *Minor crossmatch:* Mixing the donor's plasma with patient's RBCs.

Procedure (Fig. 79.1)

- Take one drop of recipient's serum/plasma in a small test tube.
- Add 5% of saline suspension of donor's RBCs
- Mix the two
- Incubate at 37°C for 1 hour
- Centrifuge
- Check for agglutination or hemolysis.

Result

Agglutination or hemolysis indicates incompatibility.

Note

- Minor crossmatch is considered as less important and not routinely performed.
- For transfusion of platelets or fresh frozen plasma, crossmatching is not required.

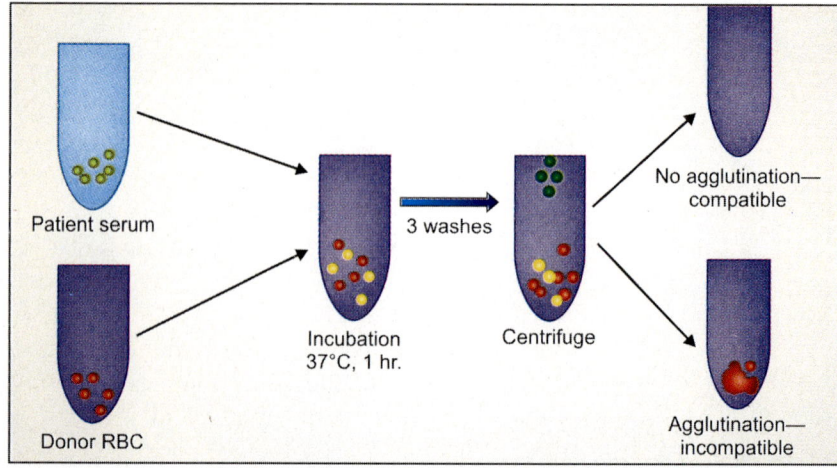

Fig. 79.1: Major crossmatch

80

Transfusion Reactions

Immediate

a. Acute hemolytic transfusion reaction
b. Febrile non-hemolytic transfusion reaction
c. Allergic reactions
d. Anaphylactic reactions
e. Transfusion related lung injury
f. Volume overload
g. Bacterial contamination.

Delayed

a. Delayed hemolytic transfusion reaction
b. Infections
c. Iron overload
d. Graft-versus-host disease
e. Post-transfusion purpura.

A. Acute Hemolytic Transfusion Reaction

- Occurs due to destruction of donor red cells by antibodies in the recipient.
- Results from transfusion of ABO mismatched blood to the recipient.
- On peripheral smear, features of hemolytic anemia are seen.
- Patient complains of fever, flank pain, increased heart rate, decrease in blood pressure.

B. Febrile Non-hemolytic Transfusion Reaction

- Most common transfusion reaction
- Patient complains of fever, chills, and increased heart rate.

C. Allergic Reaction

Second most common reported transfusion reaction.

D. Delayed Hemolytic Transfusion Reaction

- Occurs within a few days or weeks after transfusion
- Individuals are previously sensitized to red cell antigen by a previous transfusion and antibodies are present in low titers.

E. Anaphylactic Reaction

Patient presents as acute hypotension, shock, and dyspnea.

Recognition and Investigation of Transfusion Reaction

All transfusion reactions are considered as hemolytic in nature and the patient is investigated accordingly.

1. Transfusion should be immediately stopped.
2. All papers should be checked for clerical error (e.g. wrong unit given to wrong recipient).
3. Blood bank is immediately informed, and the blood bag, administration set and post-transfusion blood and urine samples should be sent to the blood bank.
4. To check for evidence of hemolysis:
   a. Peripheral smear showing features of hemolytic anemia.
   b. Hemoglobin in blood
   c. Hemoglobin in urine

Prevention of Transfusion Reactions

- Follow strictly the existing safety protocols
- Leukoreduction (blood without leukocytes) if done before transfusion, can reduce the incidence of febrile non-hemolytic transfusion reactions.
- In patients with history of allergies, transfusion of washed components is recommended, and premedication with antihistamine is done.
- In order to reduce the risk of transfusion-associated graft-versus-host disease, patient should receive the components, that have undergone prior irradiation.
- In order to avoid hypothermia, associated with large volume transfusion, warming of blood components is done.

81

Blood Components

One unit of blood can give rise to one unit of packed red cells, one unit of platelets and one unit of fresh frozen plasma/cryoprecipitate.

Whole Blood

- One unit of blood collected in 350 ml blood bag, which also contains anticoagulant (citrate phosphate dextrose adenine-1)
- It is stored at a temperature of 4–6°C
- Shelf-life is 35 days

Blood Components (Flowchart 81.1)

A. Red Cells Components

1. *Packed red cells*
   - Prepared from whole blood
   - Whole blood is centrifuged
   - Supernatant plasma is separated from red cells by transferring it to the empty bag.

Flowchart 81.1: Demonstrating component separation

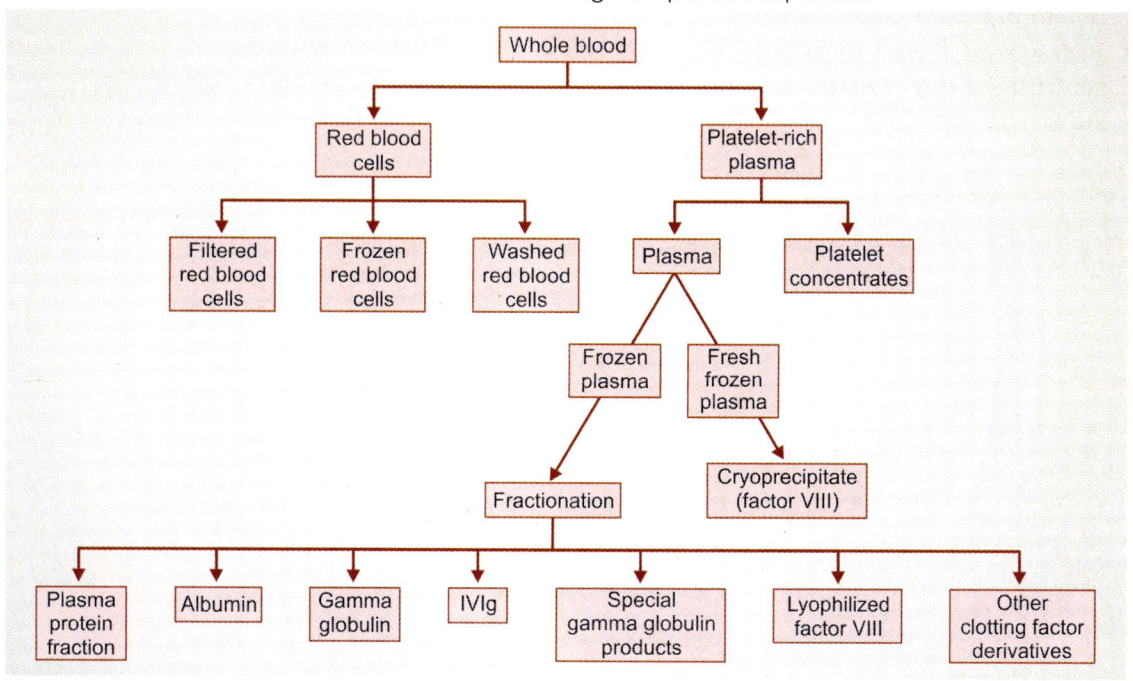

- In the primary blood bag, red cells are left behind.
- Used for patients who are anemic

2. *Leukocyte poor red cells*
   - Red cells depleted from white blood cells.
   - Reduces the risk of febrile non-hemolytic transfusion reactions.
   - Done by using leukocyte-reduction filters

3. *Washed red cells:* Red cells can be washed with normal saline.

4. *Frozen red cells*
   - Used for storage of donor RBCs
   - Frozen red cells can be stored up to 10 years

5. *Irradiated red cells*
- Gamma irradiation of RBCs inactivates lymphocytes.
- Thus, preventing the complication of graft-versus-host disease.

B. Platelets

Platelet concentrates
- One unit of whole blood is centrifuged to obtain platelet-rich plasma (PRP).
- PRP is transferred to satellite bag and is centrifuged to get platelets at bottom and supernatant plasma.

- Platelets are stored at 20–24°C with continuous agitation (in platelet agitator) and can be stored for 5 days.

C. Plasma Components

1. *Fresh frozen plasma (FFP)*
   - Prepared from whole blood within 6 hours of collection.
   - Plasma separated from platelets by centrifugation is collected into a separate bag.
   - This plasma is now rapidly frozen at −20°C.
   - FFP contains all the coagulation factors
   - It can be stored for 1 year if temperature is maintained below −25°C.
   - Before transfusion, FFP is thawed (warmed) between 30° and 37°C.
   - FFP should be transfused within 2 hours of thawing.

2. *Cryoprecipitate* contains factor VIII, von Willebrand factor, fibrinogen, factor XIII, fibronectin.

D. Plasma Derivatives

1. Human albumin
2. Factor VIII concentrate
3. Prothrombin complex concentrate
4. Immunoglobulins

Plasmapheresis

82

- Procedure by which plasma is separated from red blood cells.
- This plasma can be treated and returned or exchanged into the patient's blood circulation.
- It can be autologous (i.e. removing blood plasma, treating it and returning it to the same person) or exchange (i.e. removing the blood plasma and exchanging it with donor plasma, albumin, or albumin and saline).
- Procedure is performed outside the body and is hence called extracorporeal therapy.

Conditions for which plasmapheresis can be useful
- Guillain-Barré syndrome
- Goodpasture's syndrome
- Myasthenia gravis
- Anti-phospholipid antibody syndrome
- Hemolytic uremic syndrome
- Multiple sclerosis
- Lambert-Eaton syndrome

Can be performed by
a. Manual method
b. Automated method

83

Record Keeping in Blood Bank

Systematic procedure by which the records of an organization are created, captured, maintained and disposed off.

Record keeping includes
- Procedure of donor selection
- Collection of donated blood
- Donor screening
- Laboratory testing
- Processing and storage
- Matching and issue of blood bags for transfusion.
- Disposable system

Objectives
- To improve upon day to day work of the blood bank.
- To help promotion of voluntary blood donation.
- To provide information of donor's profile.
- To monitor availability, distribution and utilization of blood.

Standard Operating Procedures (SOPs)
- A manual should be prepared
- This manual is most important document of any blood bank system and should cover every significant action of organization.
- SOPs should be strictly followed and all procedures are performed exactly in same manner.
- SOPs ensure easy monitoring.

Specific Examples of SOP
- Donor registration and interview
- Donor selection and blood collection (phlebotomy)
- Testing of blood for transfusion transmitted infections.
- Preparation of blood components and storage.
- Quality monitoring of equipment
- Quality monitoring of laboratory techniques
- Training of staff.

84

Antibody

- Also called immunoglobulin (Ig)
- It is a large Y-shaped protein produced by the body's immune system.
- Detects the antigen in blood
- Produced by B-lymphocytes and plasma cells.
- Made up of two heavy chains and two light chains, which are composed of a variable region and constant region.

IMMUNOGLOBULINS

5 immunoglobulin classes—IgG, IgM, IgA, IgD, IgE.

Functions

a. *IgG*
  - Provides long-term protection against an infectious agent.
  - Protects against bacteria, viruses, toxins

b. *IgA*
  - Binds to the microbes before they invade tissues.
  - First defense mechanism for mucosal surfaces such as intestine, nose and lungs.

c. *IgM*
  - Involved in ABO blood group antigens on the surface of the antigens.
  - Enhance ingestion of cells by phagocytosis.

d. *IgE*
  - Binds to the mast cells and basophils, which play a role in immune response.
  - Controls parasitic infestations.

e. *IgD:* Presents on the surface of B cells and plays a role in antibody production.

Difference between IgM and IgG

See below

Feature	IgM	IgG
Structure	Pentamer	Monomer
Presence	Blood and lymph fluid	Body fluids
Antigen binding sites	Ten to twelve in number	Two
Placenta	Does not cross the placenta	Cross the placenta and can built immunity in fetus
Presence in colostrum (mother's milk)	Absent	Present
Types	One type	Four types
Onset of development of antibodies	Indicates the current infection (acute onset)	Appears after a few days of infection, when IgM is disappeared

Index

Reader's Notes

Reader's Notes